Biography of a Yogi

Biography of a Yogi

Paramahansa Yogananda and
the Origins of Modern Yoga

ANYA P. FOXEN

OXFORD
UNIVERSITY PRESS

OXFORD
UNIVERSITY PRESS

Oxford University Press is a department of the University of Oxford. It furthers
the University's objective of excellence in research, scholarship, and education
by publishing worldwide. Oxford is a registered trade mark of Oxford University
Press in the UK and certain other countries.

Published in the United States of America by Oxford University Press
198 Madison Avenue, New York, NY 10016, United States of America.

CIP data is on file at the Library of Congress
ISBN 978–0–19–066805–1 (pbk.); ISBN 978–0–19–066804–4 (hbk.)

3 5 7 9 8 6 4 2

Paperback printed by WebCom, Inc., Canada
Hardback printed by Bridgeport National Bindery, Inc., United States of America

A Yogi is a man who thinks and thinks
And never has time for forty winks,
Seldom eats, rarely drinks,
And is usually from Rangoon.

A Yogi is a man who takes a pin
And casually sticks it through his skin.
You'll always find his picture in
A "Believe It Or Not" cartoon.

With him it's mind over matter,
But I know one who lost his mind,
Became as mad as a hatter.

There was a Yogi who lost his will power.
He met a dancing girl and fell in love.
He couldn't concentrate or lie on broken glass,
He could only sit and wait for her to pass.

Unhappy Yogi, he tried forgetting,
But she was all that he was conscious of.
At night when he stretched out upon his bed of nails,
He could only dream about her seven veils.

His face grew flushed and florid
Every time he heard her name,
And the ruby gleaming in her forehead
Set his Oriental soul aflame.

This poor old Yogi, he soon discovered
She was the Maharaja's turtledove.
And she was satisfied, she had an emerald ring,
An elephant to ride and everything.

He was a passing whim.
That's how the story goes.
And what became of him,
Nobody knows.

—"THE YOGI WHO LOST HIS WILL POWER," You're the
One, 1941

Contents

Figures

Preface

THIS BOOK IS somewhat of a personal ouroboros, which is perhaps fitting given the yogic significance of coiled serpents. My first encounter with the practice that I would later come to call "modern postural yoga" occurred at the age of nineteen in the stuffy upstairs room of an unassuming office cum shopping complex in a ritzy hamlet on the Jersey Shore. Vaguely intrigued by my mother's stories of having to wring the sweat out of her clothes after class, but having almost no real idea of what "yoga" might entail, I followed her into Bikram Yoga Rumson.

I would subsequently learn that not all yoga classes were done in hundred-degree heat or left you with the kind of blissful afterglow that only emerges when one narrowly averts heat stroke. The studio I had unwittingly found myself attending was operating under the symbolic auspices of a man named Bikram Choudhury, who seemed to believe that suffering was something to be celebrated. So I suffered. And I thrived. While there are many Bikram Yoga acolytes—indeed, Bikram himself—out there with tales far more miraculous than mine, the practice fundamentally transformed my relationship with my body and in doing so transformed my life.

Yet the deeper I delved into the first kind of exercise that I had been able to sustain the more I wanted to view it as more than glorified exercise. Hoping to dispel these anxieties, I enrolled in a Hindu Philosophy class during my second year at Rutgers University, where I learned that yoga was actually about the *nirodhaḥ*-ing of *vṛtti*s rather than the doing of lunges. At the time, there was little scholarship relating modern postural practice to yoga's premodern origins and, even if this had been otherwise, it seems unlikely that I would have known where to look. Still, whatever cognitive dissonance I experienced did little to undermine my commitment to sweaty yoga classes. By the end of my junior year, I had concluded that since the economic aspect of my practice was quickly becoming unsustainable, I had better become a yoga teacher myself. That summer, I traveled to Ft. Lauderdale to study with Jimmy Barkan, one of Choudhury's oldest students and now-estranged right-hand man. I did this largely because Barkan's training was half the price of Choudhury's.

That summer I finally learned to do a push-up, decided to abandon my plan to pursue a PhD in Victorian literature, found out about the Law of Attraction, and made my first—and to this day only—vision board. I also stood on the beach every morning, fingernails loaded with sand from digging my way through seemingly endless sun salutations, and chanted into the crashing waves of the Atlantic: Mahavatar Babaji … Lahiri Mahasaya … Swami Sri Yukteswar … Paramahansa Yogananda … Bishnu Ghosh. This was our lineage. Our *parampara*. Alongside B. K. S. Iyengar's *Light on Yoga* and several works by Georg Feuerstein, we were assigned *The Autobiography of a Yogi*. I never made it to the end. Frankly, I thought it was kind of nutty. Plus, it seemed hardly more related to doing lunges than did the philosophy of the *Yoga Sūtras*.

My teacher thought otherwise. Jimmy Barkan, it turned out, was not only a student of Choudhury's postural yoga but also a spiritual disciple of Paramahansa Yogananda through the Self-Realization Fellowship. For Jimmy, these two identities were intimately connected, but only because of his own intuitive understanding on the practice. It would be a nearly a decade before I would have the opportunity to untangle with him, in a lengthy phone call, what it meant that the *āsana* practice he identified as being unique to Bishnu Ghosh's lineage was the very same one that Yogananda had taught to select American disciples. Or, even more important, why the Self-Realization Fellowship had refused to allow him to substitute the *āsana*s he had learned from Choudhury for their program's calisthenic Energization Exercises.

When I declared my desire to pursue a PhD in South Asian religions so that I could study yoga, my advisor in the English department dutifully accepted my decision but requested that I don't bring him any crystals. I was again confused. I had no idea what crystals had to do with yoga. Now I realize I was only in the dark because the resident New Ager at my teacher training had by then moved on from crystals to *The Secret*. The reason I was failing to recognize my yoga or its surrounding culture in its Indian roots was because these roots told only half of the story and perhaps not the most immediate one. Elizabeth De Michelis first sparked this idea in my mind when she called modern yoga "the graft of a Western branch onto the Indian tree of yoga."[1] I'm now inclined to modify the metaphor. Modern yoga is less a graft and more an inosculation—the place where two trees, each with their own ancient root system, have entwined so intimately that they have become one. It would take me another half a decade to figure this out.

Indeed, it was precisely when my relationship with yoga, both personally and intellectually, seemed most tenuous that the pieces finally came together. At a total loss for a dissertation topic, I sat down and finished Yogananda's *Autobiography*. Years before, I had tossed the book aside because I couldn't make sense of it. The fact is, Yogananda's work remains so difficult to place precisely because it is not any one thing. It's about yoga but not about *āsana*. It's about mystical India, but it's also about science. It's about Hinduism, but it's also about Mesmerism, Swedenborgianism, New Thought, and even Christianity. It's about a Yogi but also about a man.

The practice that drew me in, like most varieties of postural yoga in the United States, entered the mainstream during the last two decades of the twentieth century. What I did not know when I started my project was that Yogananda taught these same postures on American soil over three-quarters of a century earlier. From this perspective, they likely predate (at least in their arrival to the West) the Krishnamacaryan style that is today widely perceived to be the hallmark of modern postural yoga. Yogananda may well be the single most important figure in yoga's early American history and he marks a central turning point—from the various physical and metaphysical activities that Yogis were believed to engage in to the practice popularly known as yoga today.

As the above pages no doubt demonstrate, the journey that ended in this book has been personal at least as much as it has been scholarly. In acknowledging the many people who have made it possible, it occurs to me that I would be remiss in not starting that list with Paramahansa Yogananda himself. It is his life that has allowed me to make sense of why I keep going back to that sweaty room.

More directly, I have been fortunate in having a number of mentors who have fostered my ideas over the years. At Rutgers University, Edwin Bryant first introduced me to the classic literature on yoga as well as to South Asian religions more broadly. Whatever understanding I can claim of Indian philosophy and metaphysics, I owe to him. And although we didn't end up in the same field, I will be forever grateful to Barry Qualls for telling a panicked girl who had, in a moment of insanity, decided to take his senior seminar in her sophomore year that she wrote like an angel and then continuing to encourage her even when it meant crystals. Barbara Holdrege was my *doktormutter* in the truest sense. Without her support, both scholarly and personal, none of this would have been possible. Plus, my commas would still be a mess. David White not only offered invaluable support and insights, but his brilliant work on yoga has been central to the evolution of my own thinking. Rudy Busto filled in crucial points on the Americanist front and Catherine Albanese first introduced me to the concept of metaphysical religions.

Andrea Jain has been an invaluable mentor, colleague, and friend, who offered endless guidance on this manuscript and beyond. Philip Goldberg was not only an instrumental conversation partner but helped me to navigate the complex realities of Yogananda's living legacy. Scott Robinson, in addition to being my partner in crime for the first half of this journey, is responsible for the spark of insight that ultimately became chapter 2 of the present text. Although they were not directly involved, this book would not exist without the support of my parents, friends, and colleagues. Thanks, too, to Jimmy Barkan, my *āsana* guru.

Finally, though she'll never know it, I'd like to thank Baggins, my tiny canine muse, who slumbered peacefully on my lap as I finished the second half of this manuscript. Along with her, this book is dedicated to Brooks, my friend, partner, and basically the best person I know.

A.P.F.

Note on Transliteration

Sanskrit and other non-English terms appear in italics and are transliterated following standard lexicographics usage unless otherwise noted, with the following exceptions: (1) the term "Yogi" is used in preference to "*yogin*" whenever referring to the larger typological category; (2) terms that have entered the standard English lexicon, such as "yoga" or "guru," appear without italicization or diacritical markers; (3) Proper names are rendered without diacritical marks and follow the transliteration and spelling preferred by historical sources.

Dramatis Personae

A. K. Mozumdar, Bhagat Singh Thind, Yogi Hari Rama, Yogi Rishi Singh Gherwal, Yogi Wassan Singh, unaffiliated early twentieth-century Yogis of Indian descent

Bikram Choudhury, Hollywood Yogi superstar and founder of Bikram Yoga ("hot yoga"), disciple of Yogananda's brother, Bishnu Ghosh

Bishnu Charan Ghosh, younger brother of Yogananda, Indian physical culturalist, guru (direct teacher) of Bikram Choudhury

Helena Petrovna Blavatsky (aka Madame Blavatsky, aka HPB), Russian-born Spiritualist medium, occultist, and central founder of the Theosophical Society in 1875

Lahiri Mahasaya (b. Shyama Charan Lahiri), received Kriya Yoga doctrine from Babaji, guru of Sri Yukteswar, grand-guru of Yogananda

Mahavatar Babaji, immortal liberated being residing in the Himalayas, guru of Lahiri Mahasaya, father of Kriya Yoga

Nirad Ranjan Chowdhury (aka Sri Nerode), associate of Yogananda, 1926–1939

Pierre "The Omnipotent Oom" Bernard (b. Perry Baker), American-born Yogi, occultist, and founder of the Tantrik Order of America (1905) and Clarkstown Country Club in Nyack, New York (1918)

Sri Yukteswar (b. Priyanath Karar), disciple of Lahiri Mahasaya, guru of Yogananda

Swami Abhedananda, Swami Paramananda, early Yogis of the Vedanta SocietySwami Dhirananda (b. Basu Kumar Bagchi), childhood friend and associate of Yogananda in the United States, 1922–1929

Swami Kriyananda (b. James Donald Walters), disciple of Yogananda and founder of Ananda Church of Self Realization

Swami (Paramahansa) Yogananda (b. Mukunda Lal Ghosh), disciple of Sri Yukteswar, founder of the Self-Realization Fellowship, American Yogi extraordinaire

Swami Satyananda (b. Manamohan Mazumder), childhood friend and life-long associate of Yogananda, disciple of Sri Yukteswar

Swami Satyeswarananda, studied under Satyananda, biographer of Yogananda

Swami Vivekananda (b. Narendra Nath Datta), Indian representative at the 1893 World Parliament of Religions and one of the first Yogis to visit America, disciple of the Bengali mystic Ramakrishna, founder of Vedanta Society

Yogi Hamid Bey, Yogi Roman Ostoja, associates of Yogananda during the 1930s

Yogi Ramacharaka, pseudonym of New Thought author William Walker Atkinson

Biography of a Yogi

Introduction

THIS BOOK IS not actually a biography—at least not in the traditional sense of the word. It is not the story of a person but a persona. When Paramahansa Yogananda's *Autobiography of a Yogi* was first published in 1946, the Yogi had already become a stock character on the American cultural landscape. *Time* magazine, in a 1947 review of the then-little-known spiritual classic, provocatively titled "Here Comes the Yogiman," gives the following account of the state of things:

> Some of the most literate practitioners of the English language have written about yoga. Several of them have even sweetened their message with some of their best sex-novel tricks. But despite the literary followers of Indian philosophy—Aldous Huxley, Christopher Isherwood, John (Voice of the Turtle) Van Druten and Gerald Heard—yoga is still as mystifying as Sanskrit to the average American.
>
> One trouble is that there are no bar associations or synods to set standards among swamis (holy men, monks)—almost anyone in the U.S. can set up shop as a swami if he can find any followers. As a result, there are devout swamis who lead the good life, and there are swamis who simply enjoy a good life. Few of either kind write their autobiographies, so this life story by California's Paramhansa Yogananda (a Bengali pseudonym meaning approximately Swami-Bliss-through-Divine-Union) is something of a document. It is not likely to give the uninitiated much insight into India's ancient teachings. It does show exceedingly well how an alien culture may change when transplanted by a businesslike nurseryman from the tough soil of religious asceticism into hothouses of financial wealth and spiritual despair.

So who exactly is the "Yogiman"? And what precisely is a Yogi? Even in contemporary times, when yoga studios compete with coffee shops for the amount of real estate they take up on America's urban street corners, the Yogi remains an elusive figure.

The apprehension expressed in *Time*'s review of Yogananda's text is not an isolated incident. Early twentieth-century America was home to a flourishing lecture circuit populated by Yogis of all types. New Thought groups were a receptive audience for the recycled metaphysical teachings of career Yogis, and stage magic and "ironman" demonstrations were an equally comfortable home for Yogis and Yogi types. More important, the line between "authentic" Yogis and self-styled "imposters" was uniquely vague due to the sheer lack of information on the part of the general population. Late nineteenth- and early twentieth-century Yogis existed in a society that was simultaneously fascinated by their Oriental mystique and thoroughly ignorant of the actual details thereof. As our *Time* reviewer observes, there was no official Yogi certification program—"almost anyone in the U.S. can set up shop as a swami if he can find any followers"—which made distinguishing the genuine article, if there was such a thing, a rather murky enterprise.

On a single page of a 1930 edition of the *Los Angeles Times*, scattered in clusters among advertisements for lectures in various flavors of Christianity, we find talks by Yogananda, his recently estranged associate Swami Dhirananda, Swami Paramananda of the Vedanta Society, Bhagat Singh Thind, and Rishi Singh Gherwal. Suffice it to say, a Southern Californian with tastes more exotic than could be fulfilled by the domestic metaphysics of Christian Science and New Thought would have had no shortage of options. As Los Angeles was one of the hotbeds for Yogi activity in the pre–World War II period, one might assume that its residents would have a more cultivated palate when it came to discerning the character of these various teachers.

However, things appear to have been ambiguous enough to prompt the same *Los Angeles Times* to run an editorial titled "Who are the Swamis?" on Christmas day in 1932, the opening of which read as follows:

Who and what is a swami? According to the idea of the average person (whose information on any particular subject usually is not complete) a swami is a Hindu who wears a turban, adorns himself in colored robes, charms snakes, tells fortunes, worships idols, preaches a strange philosophy and keeps a harem.

The average person is partly right. A swami is a Hindu (Hinduism being a religion) who, when he conducts religious services, usually wears a yellow robe, which denotes spirituality and the color of his order. However, he is not interested in snake charming nor fortune telling, does not worship idols, is a believer in God, teaches the art of living and the science of becoming mentally serene, and, being an avowed celibate, never keeps a harem.

The piece profiled three local Swamis—Yogananda, Dhirananda, and Paramananda—and though the author employs the term "Swami," largely due to the fact that all three of the figures in question do belong to a monastic order and therefore make use of the title themselves, his clarification of popular opinion could have just as easily applied to the term "Yogi." Indeed, just three years prior, Yogananda published a similar passage in his *East-West* magazine under the title "Who is a Yogi?" wherein he likewise specified that a "Yogi" is "not a sword-swallower, crystal gazer or snake charmer, but one who knows the scientific psycho-physical technique of uniting the matter-bound body and soul with their source of origin, the Blessed Spirit."[1] Of course a careful reader might quickly notice that both of the above sets of statements deal not so much with what a Yogi is, but what a Yogi *does*, or does not do, as the case may be.

In the ensuing pages, I submit that what a Yogi does—or rather, the popular cultural understanding of what he does—relies on several key narrative elements or tropes. Even further, these narrative elements and tropes are in many ways the key to understanding the development of transnational postural yoga practice during the twentieth century. Specifically, we will examine the figure of the Yogi as he appears to us in the imagination of early twentieth-century America and Europe, the period that gave birth to yoga's modern-day popularity in the West. This will mean focusing both on the stories that people tell about Yogis and the dialectically related story that the Yogi tells about himself. To give grounding to what would otherwise be a very vague and scattered account, I adopt Paramahansa[2] Yogananda as a case study representative of a crucial moment in the ideological encounter between Indian and Euro-American thought and culture. The persona of the early transnational Yogi, of which Yogananda is a particular instantiation, stands at the intersection of complementary and internally conflicting narratives that draw on traditional Indian thought but simultaneously show marks of colonial and Western elements stemming from Romantic Orientalism, post-Enlightenment dialogue with popular science, and no small amount of xenophobia. By the middle of the twentieth century, these various currents would coalesce into a vision of the Yogi—and of his practice—that blended the mystical with the scientific, the particular with the universal, the body with spirit, and the human with the superhuman. And he would do much of this through what would otherwise look like good thoughts and exercise.

Chapters 1 and 2 are to a large extent parallel histories—one of agents and the other of ideas—that bring us up to speed in understanding the context in which the Yogi found himself in the first few decades of the twentieth century. Chapter 1 traces a broad history of Yogis and Yogi-figures, first contextualizing them in an Indian understanding of their identity in relation to their superhuman and superpowerful status and then moving to Western representations of the same. Chapter 2 examines the evolution of the metaphysical concepts, specifically the existence of a universal material medium, which allowed the Yogi's superpowers to become intelligible to a post-Enlightenment Western audience. The next three chapters comprise a section devoted specifically to Yogananda. Chapter 3 surveys Yogananda's life through the lens of sources other than his *Autobiography*, including alternative biographies, popular media, and community records. From there, chapter 4 analyzes Yogananda's teachings in the United States, specifically in the context of his adaptations of the *haṭha* yogic practice belonging to his lineage in light of American metaphysical sensibilities and interests and the consequent universalization of the Yogi. Finally, chapter 5 examines the *Autobiography* itself as a carefully constructed narrative of Yogananda's spiritual growth and identity as a Yogi, filtered through the lens of his audience as well as universalizing metaphysical concerns. A brief epilogue considers the case of Bikram Choudhury, the disciple of Yogananda's younger brother, Bishnu Ghosh, as an embodiment of the Yogi represented as a problematic superman before offering some final reflections.

Yoga, Yogis, and the State of their Union

It might be logical to assume that a Yogi, by definition, is one who does yoga. The Sanskrit *yogin*, at base, is just that. However, this linguistic explanation does little to clarify the term as we are then left grappling with the equally vague category of yoga itself. The last decade has seen a gradual bridging of the gap between academic scholarship on yoga, which has historically emphasized pre-modern and largely textual traditions, and the gymnastically based practice undertaken by fit white women in expensive pants that most Americans and Europeans would recognize as yoga today. Seminal studies by Joseph Alter (2004), Elizabeth De Michelis (2004), and Mark Singleton (2010) have shed light on the origins of modern yoga and its postural emphasis, while simultaneously illustrating the basic lack of strict continuity between modern postural yoga and its pre-modern counterparts. More recently, Andrea R. Jain (2014) has argued for the context-specific nature of yoga and its current status as a transnational cultural product. However, while a small number of works have shifted the focus to pre-modern Yogis, studies of modern yoga have tended to largely focus on the practice rather than on its agents.[3]

This is with good reason, since the origins and nature of yoga are hotly contested commodities. As I am writing this sentence, daily practice of *sūrya namaskār*—a popular sequence belonging to modern postural yoga also known as the sun salutation—has just been made compulsory in almost 50,000 schools, government and private, across the Indian state of Rajasthan. On the other side of the earth, the Hindu American Foundation is still nominally promoting its "Take Back Yoga" campaign, which made national news in 2010. Postural yoga, due to its rising cultural (what to say of economic) capital, has been adopted as a fundamental aspect of Hindu religious identity and touted as India's universal gift to the world.[4]

This transformation, however, would not have been possible without the very actors whose cultural specificity is now slowly disappearing into the universalist deluge that they themselves created. Alter, De Michelis, and Singleton all address Yogis insomuch as it is patently impossible to speak of the development of a practice in isolation from the individuals who developed it. However, they do so primarily in relation to activities that can on some level be recognized—or, more accurately, have come to be recognized through the processes detailed in these studies—as yoga. Yet, as we have seen from the *Los Angeles Times* editorial cited earlier, there are quite a few things that the popular imagination has conceived as being within the purview of a Yogi that have ostensibly nothing to do with yoga as such. The present study will consider these habits and practices of the Yogi and the ways in which they have shaped his image and representation in American culture.

This disjunction between the person of the Yogi and the practice of yoga is not an entirely modern phenomenon. David Gordon White circumvents (or rather subverts) this issue by referring to "descriptive 'yogi practice'" rather than "prescriptive 'yoga practice.'"[5] For White, "yogi practice" in its quintessential form entails yoking oneself to—taking over, entering into, even merging with—another, whether the other is an individual or the entire cosmos. Working from a theoretical perspective, White arrives at what is arguably the most complete possible definition of pre-modern yoga by isolating its core phenomenon:

> the yoga of yoking and the yoga of clear and luminous vision coalesced, from the time of the Vedas onward, into a unified body of practice in which yoga involved yoking oneself to other beings from a distance—by means of one's enhanced power of vision—either in order to control them or in order to merge one's consciousness with theirs. When those other beings were divine, even the absolute itself, this sort of yoking was cast as a journey of the mind across space, to the highest reaches of transcendent being.[6]

White's definition thus effectively encompasses everyone from the stock-charac-
ter Yogis of folk narratives who go around possessing unwitting victims, to world-
renouncing meditators, to cosmos-encompassing gods. At the root of the Yogi's
identity—indeed, his very being as a Yogi—is the superpower of tele-consciousness, which can manifest in all of the other tele-phenomena with which we are
now familiar: television, telekinesis, and so forth—down to an absolute conjunc-
tion with the cosmos, which White refers to as "a self-magnifying self that has
become fully realized as the 'magni-ficent' universe."[7] Lee Siegel boils down this
complex metaphysical concept to a much more familiar term: hypnotism.[8]

If Siegel's move makes the Yogi seem a bit too quotidian, consider that William
R. Pinch, in his study of armed Yogis in the medieval and (pre-)colonial period,
goes so far as to say that the distinguishing trait of the Yogi can be tied to a near-
universal definition of what it means to be "religious." He declares:

> Let us speak truth to power. There are certain universals that bind us.
> Death is one of them. We are not bound by how we choose to confront
> it. But confront it we must. And when we confront it and conquer it, we
> enter the province of religion. . . . What if the definition we settle upon
> allows wide latitude for the conjunction of religion and power? Surely such
> a definition answers the original, justifiable complaint. As the "essence"
> of religion, victory over death is precisely such a definition—because not
> only does it allow for power, it is rife with it. With death as the common
> denominator, the armed yogi is not a contradiction in terms: his conquest
> of death requires that we see him as religious, and his conquest of death
> guarantees worldly power.[9]

In the Yogi we encounter a fundamental repudiation of the only certainty that
characterizes the experience we term as human. This certainty is death, or, as a
famous skeptic who was prone to having supernatural experiences and liked to
call himself Mark Twain said, "death and taxes." To be human is to die. The Yogi is
the human who has transcended this condition. It may be due to this precise fact
that the yogic is so often conflated with the superhuman in modern popular narratives. It is also true that the Yogi's conquest of death, as a human undertaking,
is inevitably enmeshed in worldly implications, goals, and consequences. This is,
perhaps, where the taxes become relevant.

However, modern-day practitioners of yoga are neither superpowerful armed
agents (or opponents) of the state, nor are they frequently witnessed possessing
the bodies of others or, indeed, attaining immortality. What linkage then, if any,
is to be found between pre-modern and modern yoga practice if the pre-modern
occupation with immortality (bodily or otherwise) has faded into the rationalism

of physical fitness and the modern pre-occupation with sculpted bodies performing gymnastic exercises cannot be traced back further than a couple of centuries? The answer may very well lie in the identity of the Yogi—or rather in the shifts of his identity that have allowed one kind of yoga to gradually morph into another.

After all, modern postural yoga in not simply calisthenics. Or, if it is, it is often not calisthenics for their own sake. As Jain has demonstrated, postural yoga constitutes a body of religious practice in its own right.[10] The crucial shift occurs when the divinization of the body, such as it may be in a secularized context, is taken from the sphere of culturally specific esotericism and transformed into a universal human potential. Indeed, examining Yogis rather than yoga in this early period forms the crucial link between modern postural yoga and its diverse premodern heritage.

Interestingly, while the term "yoga" is recognizable to most Americans today, this would not have been the case at the turn of the century. On the other hand, as we saw earlier, "Yogi" was firmly associated with certain images and cultural stereotypes of exotic Oriental persons. For this reason, though we do find references to yoga in contemporary sources, the term is not imbued with the same cultural cachet or meaning that it carries today. Much more frequent are references to "yogi schools," "yogi philosophy," and even "yogi gymnastics," none of which necessarily share a consistent set of characteristics other than their origin in the teachings of these mysterious visitors from the mystical Orient. In this sense, modern forms of yoga practice emerge out of the intellectual work undertaken by early transnational Yogis to convert the racialized conception of the Oriental Yogi—together with his mystical philosophy and seemingly magical powers—into a universalized understanding of human psycho-somatic development and spiritual realization. In other words, the de-Orientalization of the Yogi, who is first and foremost the man with superpowers, brings about the universalization of the potentially superhuman.

Of course, to accept this argument one must first accept this definition of the Yogi. As White and Pinch have demonstrated, superhuman power—sometimes worldly, sometimes cosmic—can be seen as a constant throughout the Yogi's South Asian history. However, throughout this period the Yogi is seen as fundamentally Other. He is the lone ascetic, the tantric practitioner under the cover of night, the mercenary, the bogeyman used to scare small children. Socially speaking, Indian Yogis have always existed on the margins. Epistemologically speaking, this liminality is mirrored in their perceived identity. As Stuart Sarbacker has argued:

This teleology [of worldly power] can be termed as numinous, meaning that it is a deliberate cultivation of powers and capacities that are characteristic of a deity. Through this process, the *yogin* or *yoginī* becomes radically "other"—which is an affirmation of the salience of the comparative category of the numinous and a modification of it, as the human has become radically other. This transformation is presented in the symbolism of Indian asceticism, such as the association between the practice of yoga and the theriomorphic figure of the *nāga*, or mythic serpent.[11]

The practical reality of the Yogi's social marginalization is thus reflected in the symbolic representation or even literal understanding of him as something other than human. For Pinch, such understandings have very real political implications.[12] Even if his superpowers were mostly bunk, the Yogi could, as Pinch has argued, still be considered armed and extremely dangerous in the conventional sense. However, the aura of the superhuman, real or imagined, gave the Yogi a significant practical advantage when it came to everything from battlefield perceptions to political patronage. Thus, the Yogi's otherness and his power are historically deeply interrelated and indeed mutually dependent.

When the Yogi enters the Western imagination, he is subjected to yet another layer of othering. Such Yogis were both distillations of the varieties of Indian Yogis as well as consumable commodities or characters who played to Western assumptions about the Orient. Among them was the emaciated ascetic reclining on his bed of nails or contorted into an impossible posture along with his near-polar opposite, the turbaned magician, berobed and bejeweled. The former was to be regarded with a kind of morbid curiosity, while the latter could provide a measure of light entertainment, but both were generally reflective of a society in which worldly luxe and world-denying poverty reached absurd extremes. Both the ascetic and the magician were in their own ways unnatural to the point of appearing supernatural. The magician was more obviously so, since his trade was in things that seemed to defy the established laws of nature. The ascetic's attributed powers were subtler but ultimately no less fascinating, as Western imaginations attempted to comprehend austerities so extreme that no normal human being should be capable of them. From among their midst, however, emerged another figure: the mystic. The mystic became distinguishable from his two counterparts insomuch as his austerities, which were far more civilized, and his acts of magic, which rose above charlatanry, were seen to stem from a legitimate form of spiritual attainment. He finally found his embodiment in the figure of Swami Vivekananda, the "cyclonic monk" who, for many Americans, became the first Yogi with both a name and a voice.

Moreover, through these Western faces of the Yogi, we see the blurring of White's definition into Siegel's. Although European and American audiences had no notion of Indian metaphysics, the concomitant concepts of the transference of consciousness, or the origin of superhuman abilities, they did have something very similar. In the Yogi's case, this analogous phenomenon was most often referred to as hypnotism, though the full meaning of that term cannot be understood without reference to Mesmerism and the metaphysics of the ether, which we will examine in chapter 2. Most average Westerners, however, had no metaphysical understanding of why hypnotism worked, but they were overwhelmingly convinced that it did.

Moreover, it was increasingly believed that while one did not have to be a Yogi to practice hypnotism, it was part and parcel of the Yogi's very being to be in possession of this power. Thus, Westerners had an existing framework for interpreting the Yogi's claim to superhuman ability, and when Yogis themselves made such claims, their assertions were easily translated into a kind of mental power that their audiences could comprehend. Consequently, whatever his particular persona, the Yogi's access to and association with superpowers remained a constant even as he entered the foreign framework of the West. As we will see through the accounts of Yogis produced and consumed by Europeans and Americans, the Yogi was defined not by any practice of yoga that we would recognize as such today, but by his association with superhuman abilities and powers in one form or another.

It is worth noting that this understanding is not uniform or monolithic. Today, yoga functions as a truly transnational phenomenon and scholars focusing on the second (post–World War II) wave of yoga globalization have emphasized this quality.[13] However, at the turn of the century when the movement of both people and ideas was still far more restricted, the yoga that begins to develop in Europe and America and the yoga that is undergoing a continuing transformation in India share a more tenuous relationship. While one could certainly make the case for yoga as an emerging global phenomenon during this period, this study will focus chiefly on its importation into and development in the West where it represents a genuinely novel category worthy of specific attention. Even more precisely, as evidenced by the choice of Yogananda as a case study, our attention will chiefly be devoted to the United States. The cultural and ideological tropes and movements that surround the Yogi and his associated habits, including the emerging practice of modern postural yoga, are of course mirrored and indeed exchanged transatlantically. For instance, Mesmerism originated in France but Spiritualism in the United States and both became exceedingly popular in Britain. However, the United States developed an especially robust population of Yogis during this time period. These Yogis went on lecture tours and founded organizations, which attracted followers, which in turn garnered media attention in a way that surpassed contemporary European equivalents.

The above also begins to hint at another crucial thing that happened when actual flesh-and-blood Yogis began spreading their teachings internationally. They were forced to encounter, in its many arrangements and contexts, what historian Catherine L. Albanese has termed "metaphysical religion," a particular manifestation to the complex of ideas and practices that other scholars have identified more broadly as "occultism" or "Western esotericism."[14] This phenomenon—which forms a particularly pervasive current on the American religious landscape and is best exemplified in movements such as Spiritualism, Theosophy, Christian Science, New Thought, and most recently New Age—comprises four fundamental features: (1) the power of the mind, broadly conceived; (2) a cosmic correspondence between the mind and the world; (3) the movement of energy; and (4) salvation understood as solace, comfort, therapy, and healing.[15] As Yogis, who made their living primarily as spiritual teachers, had to interact with and accommodate the metaphysical inclinations of their audiences, their models of yoga increasingly took on a therapeutic slant insomuch as psychosomatic health was seen to be in itself salvific. Thus, as yoga was progressively portrayed as a science of health and bodily perfection that was accessible to everyone, the Yogi increasingly became a reflection of the Everyman and the Other gradually became the Self. At the hard core of yoga as religious practice, this meant that the Yogi's superhuman identity, together with his cosmic mental powers, was available to every human being. At the softer and more secular mainstream level, this resulted in a vision of yoga as a therapeutic practice targeted at the less superhuman version of the perfected body we see today.

Yet the cultural tropes that had historically identified the Yogi in the popular imagination were slow to fade away. For this reason, even Yogis who were portraying themselves as teachers of a universal spiritual system often made use of these tropes as a source of authority or even simply as marketing tactics. The image of the Yogi as mystic was the most amenable to universalization, partly because it had been constructed that way from the start. Nevertheless, elements of the ascetic and the magician continued to weave themselves into the identities of human Yogis as they navigated their new cultural landscape. In this way, the Yogi retained elements of his identity even as his powers were increasingly domesticated and rationalized.

The broader argument of this study thus traces the ways in which the essential identity of the Yogi as the man with superpowers has survived throughout history and successfully projected itself into the West through a complex process of mimesis, even as it also suggests that the mechanics of modern postural practice are a direct extension of this phenomenon. To a large extent, when individuals made the decision to aspire to be or to portray themselves as Yogis, they did so in accordance with the cultural templates that were available to them. Some of these templates were adopted subjectively, either consciously or subconsciously, while others were simply imposed on them by the outside world. However, whether the distinction at the heart of the matter is truly ontological (that is, dealing with the Yogi's state of being fundamentally Other or superhuman) or simply epistemological (dealing with the ways in which the Yogi is perceived to be superhuman) remains open to question. It is not my goal to debunk or otherwise expose Yogananda or anyone else as a spiritual charlatan or pretender. This study, for lack of a methodologically sound approach to determining the historical reality of the Yogi's superhumanity (is the Yogi *really* the man with superpowers?), will confine itself to the epistemological category of what it has meant to present oneself and to be perceived as a Yogi. That is, how and for what reasons did people take on the identity of a Yogi, and how did others in turn understand and represent them?

Some Clarifications on Terminology

A few technical details remain to be addressed. The first is one of terminology. When discussing the Yogi and his abilities, I make frequent use of words like supernatural, superhuman, and superpower(s). These are all familiar enough words, albeit the last in the sequence is more typically associated with comic book heroes than it is with spiritual adepts, especially in its plural form. When I use this latter term, as I will rather frequently throughout this work, I refer generally to some equivalent of the Sanskrit *siddhi* (and its various terminological variations such as *vibhūti, ṛddhi, labdhi*, and so on),[16] the "perfections" so ubiquitous within South Asian yogic and tantric sources. However, I have chosen to render this term in a pop cultural rather than academic register because I believe that such a translation hits closer to what is actually meant by these abilities when they are referenced both in Indian folk narratives and in Western popular media.[17] On the one hand, "superpower," in the singular and more abstract sense, refers to the extraordinary nature of the Yogi's control over his body and surrounding environment. On the other hand, "superpowers," in the more colloquially familiar form evokes the similarity between the Yogi's feats and those belonging to the superheroes of pulp fiction and comic book fame.[18]

As for the other two uses of this prefix, as in supernatural and superhuman, they too require a slight qualification. Typically, when we employ these terms in everyday language, we do so to signify something that is outside of nature, or someone who is beyond human. However, as Vivekananda reminds us, "there is no supernatural, says the Yogi, but there are in nature gross manifestations and subtle manifestations."[19] Thus "super" is used here in its meaning as "superior." The superman does not stand outside the category of man; rather, he is man at his highest potential. Man turned up to eleven, so to say. Just so, the supernatural is not herein treated as being somehow exterior to or even, strictly speaking, beyond the natural. It is nature in its highest form or degree. Thus, when these terms appear in the present study (outside of quoted passages) they are to be understood precisely in this way. To a large extent, this is because the (meta) scientific ruminations of Yogis such as Vivekananda and Yogananda necessitate such a reading. It is also, however, because the Yogi's humanity is integral to his ultimate superhumanity. The Yogi is not a god, or at least not any more so than the rest of us.

The reader will have noticed by now that I have been both rather liberal and rather ambiguous in my use of the term "Yogi." This is on many levels intentional. In part, it reflects the multivalence of Sanskrit terms that is representative of the tradition itself, which will be discussed in chapter 1. More important, however, I employ the term as a typological tool. Throughout this study, "Yogi" is used in its capitalized form specifically to signal an amalgamated category or archetype rather than to refer to any one technical use of the term (in such cases, the Sanskrit *yogin* is typically employed). Acting as a placeholder referent, it subsumes the vast multitude of historical characters—actual, fictional, and theoretical—that have lent some measure of tenuous coherence to the concept, in form even when not necessarily in name.

For instance, although Yogananda is often referred to as "Swami" due to his monastic affiliation as a renunciant, if the title of his *Autobiography* is any indication, he considered himself to be first and foremost a Yogi. In agreement with this, "Yogi" is the title almost uniformly adopted by those who sought affiliation with an aspect of its authority, from an American New Thought writer looking to establish an Oriental mystique of credibility (Yogi Ramacharaka), to a Sikh Punjabi immigrant with no formal religious training who saw a career opportunity on the metaphysical lecture circuit (Yogi Wassan), to a Borsht Belt comedian looking to distinguish himself from the pack (Mashuganishi Yogi), to a Major League Baseball player who was described by a childhood friend as sharing some mannerisms with a Indian snake charmer he had once seen on the television (Yogi Berra). The Yogi title was also adopted by two of Yogananda's more colorful associates, Yogi Hamid Bey and Yogi Roman Ostoja (both of whom we will meet in chapter 3) despite the two being, respectively, of Egyptian and Polish descent.

This study mostly concerns itself with the pre–World War II period and therefore largely does not take into account the second wave of Indian Yogis. Their teachings, and occasionally their actual persons, made their way to American shores prompted by the lifting of immigration restrictions in 1965 and the concurrent interest in Indian teachings by the international countercultural movement of the same period. In this context, "guru" becomes the term of choice and largely replaces Yogi. In his proper South Asian context, the guru is a teacher in a lineage of (often highly ritualized) practice. Thus, not every Yogi is necessarily a guru insofar as there is no obligation for the Yogi to initiate or educate others in the wisdom of his superhuman ways. I generally avoid using the term outside of cases where it represents a formal relationship between master and disciple—as in, Sri Yukteswar is the guru of Yogananda—because it rarely if ever appears in the historical sources of this earlier period, which overwhelmingly prefer "Yogi," "Swami," or occasionally "fakir."[20]

The Context of Orientalism and the "West"

A similarly amalgamating critical move has recently been made by Jane Iwamura in her study of a phenomenon she identifies as "Virtual Orientalism," which she sees manifested in the figure of the Oriental Monk onto whom we project our assumptions, fears, and hopes. She argues:

> Although the Oriental Monk has appeared to us through the various media vehicles of American pop culture, we recognize him as the representative of an otherworldly (though perhaps not entirely alien) spirituality that draws from the ancient wellsprings of "Eastern" civilization and culture. . . . The term Oriental Monk is used as a critical concept and is meant to cover a wide range of religious figures (gurus, bhikkus, swamis, sifus, healers, masters) from a variety of ethnic backgrounds (Japanese, Chinese, Indian, Tibetan). Although the range of individual figures points to a heterogeneous field of encounter, all of them are subjected to a homogenous representational effect as they are absorbed by popular consciousness through mediated culture. Racialization (more correctly, "orientalization") serves to blunt the distinctiveness of particular persons and figures. Indeed, the recognition of any Eastern spiritual guide, real or fictional, is predicated on his conformity to general features that are paradigmatically encapsulated in the icon of the Oriental Monk: his spiritual commitment, his calm demeanor, his Asian face, his manner of dress, and—most obviously—his peculiar gendered character.[21]

Orientalism has, of course, been popularized as a critical category by Edward Said's famous 1978 work of the same name, in which he defines it as "the corporate institution for dealing with the Orient—dealing with it by making statements about it, authorizing views of it, describing it, by teaching it, settling it, ruling over it: in short, Orientalism as a Western style for dominating, restructuring, and having authority over the Orient."[22] Whereas Said's exempla are drawn primarily from the Middle East, Iwamura's mostly swing to the Far East, but neither captures appropriately the specificity of elements construed as South Asian. Iwamura sees the Oriental Monk as coming to ascendance after World War II when images of evil Fu Manchus and the Yellow Peril are replaced with "friendlier, more subservient" models,[23] with only a brief nod to the Transcendentalists and the 1893 World Parliament of Religions. However, a look at the prewar period reveals a different yet equally complex picture. Iwamura's Oriental Monk with his spiritual enlightenment can perhaps be seen as the culmination—or the further Orientalist dilution—of the mystic Yogi, who ultimately reigns supreme in cultural longevity over his more exotic counterparts.

Accounts of the time period in question largely bear out a treatment of the Orient as a single mass entity. A pseudo-sociological study published by Harold R. Isaacs in 1958 makes the following elucidating remark:

> Hardly anything marks more clearly the limits of the American world outlook than the official and popular acceptance of the term "East–West struggle" to describe our conflict with Russia. It suggests how unthinkingly we can still accept the notion that "East" means Eastern Europe, how truly dim and undefined the farther "East" really is, how unblinkingly we give currency to a term that cuts us off psychologically from the "East" and allows Russia so much more easily to identify with it.[24]

Thus, if in the 1950s, Russia was still commonly construed as the East, then it is not at all surprising that the Russian expatriate Helena Blavatsky would have had no trouble laying claim to an Oriental exoticism when founding the Theosophical Society over three-quarters of a century earlier in 1875. It is even less surprising that Americans of the same period would have been virtually unable to distinguish between South Asians, Middle Easterners, and North Africans, especially once a turban was involved. While Isaacs found that his subjects, slightly more than half of whom had had some professional involvement with Asia and Asian affairs, did have a slightly better sense of China than they did of India, they nevertheless characterized both nations in terms of extreme Otherness, either racial or religious. Many kinds of people inevitably bled together into a single foreign sea of humanity, as his subjects gave impressions of dark skin, strange customs, different languages, different minds, different morals, different souls.[25]

Unlike British and French Orientalism, however, American Orientalism was not accompanied by a colonial project and thus took on a slightly different tenor than these European varieties. According to anthropologist Milton

Singer, "Americans tended to take over and exaggerate … the prevailing European images of India."[26] In other words, being further removed from the physical realities of the Indian subcontinent allowed Americans an even greater freedom of imagination when it came to imposing their imagined narratives onto India and its people. Orientalism thus has served not simply as an imperializing force but also as a wellspring of internal narratives. A prime example of this phenomenon is Sheldon Pollock's analysis of German Orientalism as constructive of nationalistic Aryan-race ideology.[27] The Germans, who likewise had no significant political or economic stake in India, effected a colonialism that was ideological rather than physical in nature. This results in an introverted Orientalism wherein texts of the Other are used in positive manner to elevate the Self. In a similar dynamic, on American soil, Orientalism combined with the ideologies of a universal religion allowed the West to claim India's holy men as its own. The superhuman potential of the Yogi becomes the latent birthright of all humanity.

Of course, not all Americans saw the sudden influx of Indian ideas and, in smaller doses, Indian people as a culturally elevating phenomenon. In analyzing the multivalent nature of Indian Orientalism, Richard King has pointed out that perspectives easily became polarized depending on context. Underscoring the importance of charismatic celebrities like Vivekananda in reshaping the Orientalist thought, King observes:

> In Vivekānanda's hands, Orientalist notions of India as "other worldly" and "mystical" were embraced and praised as India's special gift to humankind. Thus the very discourse that succeeded in alienating, subordinating and controlling India was used by Vivekānanda as a religious clarion call for the Indian people to unite under the banner of a universalistic and all-embracing Hinduism.[28]

Thus the Orient, even pre-Vivekananda, was characterized by a sharply bipolar nature. On the one hand, it served as a receptacle of Western fear and disgust at its purported uncivilized backwardness and depravity. On the other, it was a place of a kind of magic, mystery, and spiritual enchantment that had long faded from the rationalist landscape of Western culture.[29] The same general framework could be applied to the Yogi, who for some came to represent everything that was depraved and backwards about India, while for others stood as the embodiment of spirituality and human potential. The Yogi was grotesque yet fascinating in his mortifications, deceitful yet enchanting in his magic tricks, and, above all, visionary and venerated yet sinister and threatening in his hypnotic powers.

A Note on Gender and Sexuality

It is hardly necessary to state that the Yogi is, essentially by default, male. Historically, descriptive texts speak of Yogis as male and prescriptive manuals almost uniformly assume a male body. The female counterpart of the Yogi does exist of course. She is the *yoginī*. However, unlike the Yogi who literally embodies the bridge from human to superhuman, she is almost always more of a mythological creature, sometimes with animalistic features, than she is a human woman.[30] Although there is a small but dense body of scholarship on the roles that women have played (and not played) in yoga practice,[31] the fact remains that until very recently yoga has been a man's world. For our purpose, it can be safely stated that virtually all the images of Yogis that found their way into the West leading up to the twentieth century were images of men. To be more specific, they tended to be highly crafted images of racialized men.

The Indian Yogi also finds himself at the center of a complex web of sexuality. In some cases, it is a ritualized sexuality that essentially defines him as a Yogi, insomuch as certain systems of medieval tantric practice were based on the transmutation of sexual fluids into the elixir of immortality by virtue of which the Yogi ascended to his superhuman status.[32] More broadly, the Yogi's presumed celibacy was often seen to be a contributing factor to his superpowers, insomuch as many Indian systems of thought associate seminal retention with energetic potency. In reconciling the Yogi's sexuality, as Alter has noted, it would be quite convenient to simply state that "yoga is as Maha Yogi does"[33] and conclude that the Yogi's sexuality is easily resolved in the paradox embodied by Śiva, the paradigmatic divine Yogi and the famous erotic ascetic.[34] In real life, however, human Yogis are not always as proficient at embodying the perfect tension of the paradox as their divine model. Indeed, many Indian narratives turn on the character of the licentious Yogi or the superpowerful Yogi tempted by women both human and divine. Thus, even when not typologized as "sexy" by conventional standards—a distinct point of divergence between perceptions of pre-modern Yogis and modern-day yoga practitioners—it appears that, throughout his history, the Yogi has inevitably possessed a sexual potency that both makes him imposing and occasionally gets him into trouble.

Unsurprisingly, this becomes an issue for turn-of-the-century Euro-American sensibilities. Robert G. Lee has argued, though referring primarily to East Asians, that amidst the Victorian calcification of dimorphic gender, "Oriental sexuality was construed as ambiguous, inscrutable, and hermaphroditic; the Oriental (male or female) was construed as a 'third sex.' "[35] This is to a large extent true insomuch as Yogi-figures are often portrayed in popular discourse in a rather paradoxical fashion as being interchangeably feminine and hyper-masculine.

Such representations can generally be organized according to the following paradigm: Yogis may tend to be feminine in appearance (as descriptions often linger on their long flowing hair, soft dark eyes, and so forth), but this gentle exterior belies a hyper-masculine and even predatory sexuality. Moreover, this sexuality is inextricably tied to the Yogi's superhuman power. Female disciples—disaffected and otherwise—frequently describe being drawn to the mysterious spiritual power of their teachers. On the other hand, in a predictable turn of perspective, critics attribute this phenomenon to a malicious hypnotic influence. In this sense, the Yogi's power, real or imagined, once again becomes fundamental to his identity.

Positioning Yogananda

One last question thus remains: why Yogananda? I must admit that the general lack of scholarship on him is still somewhat of a mystery to me. Yogananda has thus far received little attention in studies of modern yoga because what he taught does not look to us like yoga. The reality, as this study will demonstrate, is that Yogananda's method as it is still taught by the Self-Realization Fellowship is essentially *haṭha* yoga par excellence due to its inherent logic of energy but has been excluded from histories of modern yoga because it largely lacks *āsanas* (postures). However, to put things into perspective, though Vivekananda is often hailed as the father of modern yoga,[36] his brand of yoga resembles modern practice even less than Yogananda's. Others have recently nominated Americans like Pierre Arnold Bernard and Ida Craddock for the title.[37] Suffice it to say that yoga's paternity remains a rather ambiguous matter.

While I have no intention to plead Yogananda's case as the authentic yoga patriarch, I do wish to nominate him as the best exemplum of an early Western Yogi that history can give us. He was certainly not the first. That title probably goes to Vivekananda. Nor was he the only. There are many other Yogis—foreign and domestic in origin—that dot the American landscape of the early twentieth century. However, he represents a unique constellation of characteristics: Indian origins (and lineage) combined with half a lifetime spent in America; a modern practice grounded in physical culture combined with *haṭha* yogic metaphysics; a groomed mystic exterior combined with stints on the vaudeville circuit; and, finally, a legacy of practice that survives to the present day.

Mark Stephens credits Yogananda with creating the very first American yoga "brand"—his Yogoda method—which he nevertheless describes as "primarily bhakti and raja and very little Hatha."[38] Meanwhile, Shreena Gandhi briefly mentions that "the figure and philosophies of Paramahansa Yogananda best embodies the guru of the 1920s, 30s, 40s & 50s."[39] However, although Yogananda makes cameo appearances in a number of studies ranging from the impact of New Thought[40] on early American yoga to anti-Asian immigration legislation,[41] there has yet to be a sustained study that addresses his impact on the landscape of modern yoga. To date, the only scholarly work of which I am aware that engages Yogananda and his legacy in a non-tangential way is Lola Williamson's work on the Self-Realization Fellowship as one among three groups that she classifies as "Hindu-Inspired Meditation Movements" (HIMMs).[42] However, Yogananda is not the sole focus of Williamson's work, which is a historically situated ethnography of three HIMMs. She draws largely on sanctioned biographical sources, including Yogananda's own *Autobiography* as well as those of his Self-Realization Fellowship (SRF)-affiliated associates. As such, Yogananda's biography, although presented in a historical manner, appears in a heavily redacted and limited form.

Leaving aside Vivekananda, whose direct impact is mitigated by the fact that he spent only about five years on American soil,[43] Yogananda is the only early Yogi to withstand the test of time. Unlike other men whose legacies now survive only in a couple of out-of-print publications and the genealogical probings of their grandchildren, Yogananda has left behind a living legacy. His SRF organization boasts five hundred centers and meditation groups worldwide. These figures do not account for any persons affiliated with splinter groups, the most prominent of which is the Ananda Church of Self Realization, led by Yogananda's direct disciple, Swami Kriyananda.[44] In any case, these figures are fairly modest, as far as popular influence is concerned. Yogananda's real claim to fame is his celebrated *Autobiography of a Yogi* (1946), which has sold over four million copies and been translated into thirty-three languages.[45] I suspect that the actual number of readers reaches far beyond this because it is the kind of book that people lend to others.

To put it simply, then, Yogananda survives in the public imagination for one main reason: he told a good story. His *Autobiography*—which is really, to borrow a term coined by Robin Rinehart, an auto-hagiography[46]—is a multifaceted portrait of the Yogi. In this sense, it is telling that the vast majority of the book takes place in India and well more than half of it details events in which Yogananda has no direct involvement. As such, the chief message of the *Autobiography of a Yogi* is the Yogi's categorical enmeshedness in the existences of other Yogis. The figure of the Yogi is constructed out of a cacophony of individual plots that represent particular human instantiations of one superhuman ideal.

More concretely, Yogananda is a crucial figure in the history of modern yoga because he stands at the fascinating intersection of reimagined Indian spirituality and Western metaphysical thought in a way that Vivekananda never did, if only because of his sustained presence in the United States. The end of Yogananda's life also corresponds with two key developments on the American metaphysical scene: first, the emergence of the New Age movement and, second, the shift from more metaphysically based and holistic under-standings of yoga to the mass popularization of postural practice. From a his-torical viewpoint, the *Autobiography* thus serves as an important artifact of this period if one seeks to construct a history of ideas. However, Yogananda's *Autobiography* is also significant because it is precisely that—the Yogi's own story. Although we have many records of others representing and interpret-ing the figure of the Yogi, we have far fewer records of the Yogi representing and interpreting himself, especially in as sustained a way as Yogananda's self-portrait presents to us. Thus, Yogananda's work provides a unique opportunity to glimpse the construction of the Yogi as he himself effects it.

From a cultural perspective, if one has any remaining doubts as to Yogananda's significance, one has only to take a look at the album cover of the Beatles' 1967 *Sgt. Pepper's Lonely Hearts Club Band*, which is a kind of "Where's Waldo?" game for Yogananda's lineage, featuring Yogananda as well as his guru Sri Yukteswar, his guru's guru Lahiri Mahasaya, and even something that looks very much like the upper half of the head of the great Mahavatar Babaji himself. George Harrison apparently keeps stacks of the book around his house to hand out to people who "need a bit of regrooving."[47] Apple founder Steve Jobs allegedly re-read it yearly and had it distributed at his memorial service in 2013.[48] However, while Yogananda has gone down in popular history as one of the great spiritual masters of the twentieth century, a closer look at his life reveals a much more compli-cated story. It is this story that I will seek to contextualize and explore in the present study.

I

The Turbaned Superman

*Let us not, however, turn away from the yogi with contemp-
tuous indifference on account of his preposterous pretensions,
for naked, emaciated, and covered with ashes though he be, he
represents, albeit in an unhealthy form, an important idea.
In the groveling world of polytheistic India, he stands forth a
bold and ever-present asserter of man's inherent dignity and
exalted position in the universe. Before the multitude cowering
in abject terror at the altars of hideous and terrible idols, he
appears as an embodiment of the belief that man, even though
he be degraded and trammeled by his fleshly garment, can by
his own exertions raise himself to divine heights of knowledge
and power.*

—JOHN CAMPBELL OMAN, *Indian Life: Religious and Social*

WHERE ONE BEGINS a history of the Yogi naturally depends on what—or
whom—one recognizes as falling into this semantic domain. In turn-of-the-
century America, the figure of the Yogi predictably becomes a canvas onto
which Western fantasies and fears are imposed with occasionally caricatured
effect. Of course, these emotions along with their accompanying representations have a history, both foreign and domestic. While early Western impressions of Yogis found in travelers' and missionary accounts are inevitably murky
visions drawn up by outsiders attempting to make sense of an often impen-
etrable social order, even a funhouse mirror offers some semblance of the
original. As the voices of actual flesh-and-blood Yogis enter the conversation,
they overwhelmingly do so along the lines of an already established script that
reflects the assumptions and expectations of their audiences. Yogi figures idealized as ascetics, magicians, and eventually mystics form the patterns for these
interpretations.

Indian Yogis have historically been a diverse group, not only because practitioners have disagreed over what constitutes "proper" yoga but also because
popular understandings of who Yogis are and what they do have refracted these

disagreements into an ever more complex mosaic. Thus, what a Yogi is depends largely on whom you ask.

For example, John Campbell Oman, Professor of Natural Sciences at Government College in Lahore and author of several pseudo-ethnographic works on Indian society and culture, observed in 1903:

> *Yogi* properly means one who practices *yoga* with the object of uniting or blending his soul with the Divine Spirit or World-Soul. . . . Very curiously, however, the practice of *yoga* is not undertaken by all *Yogis*, nor is it confined to the professed *Yogi*. The efficacy of the system is an article of faith so universally accepted throughout India, that other sectarians, including laymen, even married men and householders, resort to it when so inclined.[1]

In Oman's statement, we begin to see the emergence of a universalized yoga as a meditative and ultimately salvific process that is simultaneously open to every human being and not directly associated with its etymologically affiliated agent, the Yogi himself. The fact that Campbell is able to claim that not all Yogis practice yoga signals a widening gulf between the Yogi's eclectic identity and the increasingly metaphysical nature of the practice of yoga. Oman is ultimately ambiguous about the association between yoga and his identification of the Yogi, whom he views as an ascetic belonging to a specific suborder of Śaivism. He was writing at a time when the philosophical system of the *Yoga Sūtras*, lifted up by Orientalists as exemplary of yoga in its pure forms and codified as a universalistic "Raja Yoga" by Vivekananda, was quickly gaining in prominence.[2] It is worth noting, however, that even the *Yoga Sūtras*—that bastion of classical meditative philosophy— devotes the entire length of one of its four chapters to superpowers.

The clean cerebral universalism of yoga thus stands in direct opposition to the chaotic narratives of Yogis and their ilk, often dirty, contorted, deceitful, and occasionally armed to the teeth. Pinch, in examining premodern European accounts of Yogis, observes:

> Sixteenth and seventeenth-century authors tended to speak of *yogis* (or *jogi, ioghee*) when describing these kinds of men, sometimes in a disparaging manner. The eighteenth century saw the increased use of terms *sanyasi* (*sannyasi, sunnasee*) and *fakir* (*faquir, fukeer*), particularly by British officials in Bengal. To the west, toward Allahabad, Lucknow, and Delhi, the term *gosain* (*gossye, gusain, gusaiyan*) prevailed. Further west still, towards Jaipur in particular, the terms *bairagi* (*byragee, vairagi*) gained prominence).[3]

This assortment of terminologies is clearly regionally inflected and undoubtedly reflects what was probably an extremely complicated social structure of various sects with at times conflicting interests. In popular representations, the descriptions and images of these groups largely melded together, with Yogi and Fakir (often pronounced as "faker") emerging as the most commonly used terms in nineteenth-century and early twentieth-century America. The twentieth century would see both of these terms nearly eclipsed by "Swami" due to the strong public presence of Vedanta Society monks (taking up the organizational mantle established by Vivekananda) and other figures like Yogananda who used the title.

However, even when Americans gained access to Yogis in the flesh, foreign sights did not fail to capture the imagination. When Robert Ripley, founder of the famous "Believe it or Not!" franchise, visited India to collect oddities for the 1933–1934 Century of Progress Exposition in Chicago, he was expressly interested in "ascetics and fakirs, men who hold up their arms, sit on beds of nails, gaze at the sun, hang upside down, etc."[4] In turn, American Yogis, especially those who could not easily erase their exoticism due to being non-Western in origin, often capitalized on the perceived strangeness with which their personas were associated even as they overwhelmingly pushed a Westernized universalistic spirituality.

Premodern Yogis

Questions of identity are complicated by the fact that the Yogis whom self-proclaimed members of the tribe, like Yogananda, idealize are entirely different from the Yogis whom they describe anecdotally and after whom they model their behavior. For Yogananda, as for Vivekananda and indeed for most neo-Hindu and modern metaphysical proponents of yoga, the prototypical Yogi is the Vedic *ṛṣi* (often Anglicized in modern sources as "Rishi") or seer.

From a purely typological perspective, the *ṛṣi* may certainly be identified with the general category of the Yogi. *Ṛṣi*s feature prominently in the Ṛg Veda, an ancient text tied to India's Brāhmaṇical ritual tradition, where they are portrayed as divine or semi-divine beings who are "friends and companions to the gods, conversing with them about truths and assisting them in their creation and maintenance of the cosmic order."[5] The *ṛṣi*s are not only able to cognize the basic material and origins of the cosmos but are in fact complicit in the act of creation and the revelation of cosmic truths. This role, which is characterized by the most fundamental model of superpower insofar as it intimately associates its agent with the workings of the cosmos, is maintained throughout later epic and Purāṇic sources.

There is a measure of historical—rather than simply thematic—accuracy to the association of the *ṛṣi* and the Yogi, insofar as Vedic discourse, authored by the brahmin priestly social class, often coopted the language of martial power that belonged to the ruling *kṣatriya* class. Thus, the brahmins, who were after all believed to be the human representatives and descendants of the semi-divine *ṛṣis* and whose power rested in their control over the ritual recitation of Vedic hymns, were able to ideologically weave themselves into the system of political power by linking their ritual orality to martial conquest and applying to the former the discursive register of the latter. According to White, it was precisely this association that led to the first fundamental schism in the historical understanding of yoga, stemming from a parting of the ways in both the means and the goals of "yogic" practice starting in the third or fourth century of the Common Era:

> On the one hand, there is the practice of yoga, which leads to supernatural enjoyments and visionary "embodied" travel to the highest worlds, followed by a deferred final liberation at the end of a cosmic eon; on the other, there is meditation on the absolute, which leads directly to release from suffering existence and a disembodied identity with the godhead. The former carries forward the traditions of the yogic apotheosis of the chariot warrior, while the latter, which is clearly on the ascendant, is an adaptation of the visionary yoga of the vedic poets.[6]

White juxtaposes the yoga of the Vedic seers, based on knowing, with the yoga of the Vedic warriors, based on going.[7] The *ṛṣis* were, of course, "knowers" par excellence. It was they who first cognized the eternal Vedic hymns, which are tied to the very fabric of creation. The *kṣatriya*s, on the other hand, aspired not so much to mystical cognition as to a bodily apotheosis that accompanied the battle field death of an accomplished warrior. White relies of the Vedic meaning of yoga as "rig"—functioning as both a noun and a verb—to argue for its applicability to the literal ascent of the fallen hero into celestial realms. So historically the *ṛṣis* were indeed metaphorical Yogis but it is only after this paradigm shift in the meaning of "yoga" and the internalization of apotheosis that they become the literal model.

This disjunction also parallels a distinction between the worldly model of the *jīvanmukta* (liberated while living) and the transcendent state of *videhamukti* (liberated after death), or embodied and disembodied liberation. Stuart Sarbacker has quite elegantly expressed this in his typology of "numinous" and "cessative" models of yogic practice that span across Hindu, Buddhist, and Jain systems.[8] Whereas the cessative aspect refers to those segments of yogic practice that seek to extricate the practitioner from worldly existence, the numinous models deal with the ways in which attainment manifests in the context of worldly experience. And the ways in which it manifests is generally through superpowers. It is important to note that these superpowers are pervasive throughout the history of yogic practice and are not specific to any one tradition.[9] This distinction remains relevant even when one examines the importation of yoga into the West and its subsequent representations in the Western imagination. The same distinction, however, oftentimes blurs when one examines on-the-ground realities of flesh-and-blood Yogis. The relationship between Yogis who exhibit superpowers and Yogis who represent themselves as detached beings seeking enlightenment is often much more problematic than such a neat division would suggest.

Although the cessative mode of yoga certainly factors into historical representations of common Yogi practice, the numinous mode (or suggestions thereof) is understandably more, so to speak, visible. After all, while disembodied enlightenment is rather difficult to describe with any degree of accuracy, evidence of worldly attainment is both easier and more entertaining to discuss and represent. It should be noted, of course, that the two are not mutually exclusive.

Yogic superpowers are most fully elaborated within the tantric corpus, the beginnings of which can be traced to roughly the sixth century of the Common Era. This is also perhaps the closest that we get to an "insider" perspective on the practices of the would-be Yogi. Rather than descriptive accounts by outsiders, tantric texts are generally prescriptive manuals on how to be, or begin to become, a Yogi.

Most medieval tantric texts deal quite freely with the reality of yogic superpowers. Furthermore, when we encounter power-oriented forms of tantric practice, whether in the context of Śaiva, Vaiṣṇava, or Buddhist traditions, they are fully integrated into the soteriological systems of their respective context. Meaning, medieval tantric practitioners generally saw no contradiction between the pursuit of worldly power and the quest for liberation.[10] Such descriptions of superpowers even pervade Islamicized variants of yogic traditions and practices.[11] Texts often provide vast catalogs of powers, even going so far as to classify them hierarchically, sometimes in correlation with the *guṇas*, the three constituents of primordial matter. Superior *siddhis*, or superpowers, include providing aid in cases of disaster, conquering death, eloquence and poetic talent, sovereignty of all the worlds, and achieving final liberation. Intermediate *siddhis*, or "white magic," are generally more Machiavellian in character and include subjugating others to one's will, attracting others (especially, and perhaps unsurprisingly, women), flying, and making oneself invisible. Inferior *siddhis* represent the domain of "black magic" and include murder; rendering one's victim dumb, deaf, or blind; and altering one's form. The eight traditional *siddhis* are variously placed among this hierarchy of categories.[12]

Tantric systems of practice, regardless of sectarian affiliation, largely share the character of a ritual framework aimed at purifying—often through literally or symbolically deconstructing—the adept's body and ritually reconstituting it as a perfected body composed of *mantra* powers, at which point one may be considered a *siddha*, or perfected being. The "ground zero" of tantric practice is the body of the individual male practitioner, which is subjected to a variety of ritual activities aimed at a range of different aims. The terminology applied to this practitioner is similarly variable. The most consistent subject of the manuals' prescriptions is the *sādhaka*, or the adept. Within the southern Śaiva Siddhānta and Vaiṣṇava Pāñcarātra traditions, the *sādhaka* is the third of four possible stages in a hierarchy of initiated practitioners. Having undergone two sets of ritual initiations, he has chosen the path of worldly powers as his ultimate goal. However, while the Śaiva Āgama texts regularly use the term *sādhaka* synonymously with *yogin*, other texts take pains to distinguish the *sādhaka* from his otherwise superpowerful counterparts.

For instance, the *Jayākhya Saṃhita*, an authoritative Pāñcarātra text, insists that, unlike the *yogin* or the *tapasvin*, whose power derives from an accumulated store of practice that can be depleted by use, the power of the tantric *sādhaka* is more permanent. Although his practice involves a wide range of acts that follow the standard repertoire of tantric ritual (ritual purification, imposition of *mantras*, visualization, internal and external worship, and so forth), the heart of the *sādhaka*'s efforts is in the control of *mantra*, and all of the *sādhaka*'s oblations, recitations, and meditations are aimed at acquiring control of a particular *mantra* deity.[13] Once "conquered," the *mantra* deity (which normally appears anthropomorphically) is under the *sādhaka*'s full and permanent control and cannot be lost or depleted. This allows him to use to his heart's content the attendant powers, which cover the typical range of immortality, flight, being obscenely attractive to women, and so forth.[14] Thus, unlike more discrete rituals of magic that are geared at particular results, the *sādhaka* becomes intrinsically superpowerful. It should be added that, unlike the *tapasvin, saṃnyāsin*, and the rest of the superpower-possessing cohort, the *sādhaka* is also not conceived of as a reclusive renunciant. He remains a part of his human community and is indeed expected to use his power and authority for the benefit of others as well as himself.

However, given that such terminological distinctions do not appear to be universal even within the tantric corpus, we can perhaps cautiously identify the tantric *sādhaka* with the popular Yogi, while at the same time taking to heart the special nature of his superpowers. To this end, Hélène Brunner has proposed that the *sādhaka* is ultimately an ambiguous sort of figure who combines the features of the classical *yogin*—that is, his solitary introverted practice and the power and potential liberation that arise from it—and the popular magician who is seen as the purveyor of spells and concoctions aimed at far more practical ends.[15]

In addition to their semi-divine counterparts—whether Vedic ṛṣis or tantric siddhas—Yogis did also have corresponding divine models. Śiva, often called Mahāyogi, is the ascetic Yogi in prototype. Indeed, the renunciants of many Śaiva sects model their appearance in imitation of Śiva. Krishna, a favorite model of Yogananda, also has considerable Yogi credentials to his name and exhibits considerable Yogi-like powers, in addition to his rather orthodox discourse on yoga in the Bhagavad Gītā. However, as White concludes:

> The question—of whether the innovators of the new theism were theorizing their respective deities' omnipotence and omnipresence in terms of powers already attributed to yogis, or whether the theorization of the omnipotence and omnipresence was modeled after the attributes of the gods—remains an open one.[16]

For our purposes, the question of which came first may not be ultimately significant. Much more relevant is the association of yogic superpower with essentially divinized, cosmic states. In this sense, the Yogi serves as a literal bridge between human and divine.

Colonial Yogis

Western accounts of Yogis go as far back as Alexander the Great's encounters with the Indian gymnosophists, or "naked philosophers," during his military campaign beginning in 326 BCE. Jumping forward to the fourteenth century of the Common Era, we have accounts from Marco Polo, who spoke of Kashmiri conjurers who could "bring on changes of weather and produce darkness, and do a number of things so extraordinary that no one without seeing them would believe them." We also have the account of Ibn Battuta, a Moroccan traveler and guest of the emperor of Delhi, who describes two rather interesting Yogis, one of whom turned into a levitating cube and another who levitated a sandal.[17]

In such depictions, Yogis, fakirs, and traveling magicians become largely conflated as the performers of all manner of apparently superhuman tricks. Accounts by European merchants and travelers during the sixteenth, seventeenth, and early eighteenth centuries— including Ludovico di Varthema, Pietro della Valle, Duarte Barbosa, Ralph Finch, Jean-Baptiste Tavernier, John Fryer, Jean de Thevenot, Giovanni Francesco Gamelli Careri, and François Bernier[18]—paint a consistent if chaotic picture. Various spellings of "Yogi" are found throughout their accounts, along with other related terms. Bernier's seventeenth-century account is particularly enlightening:

> Among the vast number and countless variety of *Fakires*, or *Derviches*, and *Holy Men*, or *Gentile* hypocrites of the *Indies*, many live in a sort of convent, governed by superiors, where vows of chastity, poverty, and submission are made. So strange is the life led by these votaries that I doubt whether my description of it will be credited. I allude particularly to the people called *Jauguis*, a name which signifies "united to God." Numbers are seen, day and night, seated or lying on ashes, entirely naked. . . . Some have hair hanging down to the calf of the leg, twisted and entangled into knots, like the coat of our shaggy dogs . . . I have seen several who hold one, and some who hold both arms, perpetually lifted above the head; the nails of their hands being twisted, and longer than half my little finger, with which I measured them. . . . I have often met, generally in the territory of some *Raja*, bands of these naked *Fakires*, hideous to behold. Some had their arms lifted up in the manner just described; the frightful hair of others either hung loosely or was tied and twisted round their heads; some carried a club like to Hercules; others had a dry and rough tiger skin thrown over their shoulders. . . . Others again I have observed standing steadily, whole hours together, upon their hands, the head down and the feet in the air. I might proceed to enumerate various other positions in which these unhappy men place their body, many of them so difficult and painful that they could not be imitated by our tumblers. . . . Some of the *Fakires* enjoy the reputation of particularly enlightened saints, perfect *Jauguis*, and really united to God. They are supposed to have renounced the world, and like other hermits they live a secluded life in a remote garden, without ever visiting town. When food is brought to them, they receive it: if none be offered to them it is concluded that the holy men can live without food, that they subsist by the favour of God, vouchsafed on account of previous long fasts and other religious mortifications. Frequently these pious *Jauguis* are absorbed in profound meditation. It is pretended, and one of the favoured saints himself assured me, that their souls are often rapt in an ecstasy of several hours' duration; that their external senses lose their functions; that the *Jauguis* are blessed with a sight of God, who appears as a light ineffably white and vivid, and that they experience transports of holy joy, and a contempt of temporal concerns that defy every power of description.
>
> . . .
>
> I have now to give an account of certain *Fakires* totally different from the *Saints* just described, but who also are extraordinary personages. They

almost continually perambulate the country, make light of everything, affect to live without care, and to be possessed of the most important secrets. The people imagine that these favoured beings are well acquainted with the art of making gold, and that they prepare mercury in so admirable a manner that a grain or two swallowed every morning must restore a diseased body to vigorous health, and so strengthen the stomach that it may feed with avidity, and digest with ease. This is not all: when two of these good *Jauguis* meet, and can be excited to a spirit of emulation, they make such a display of the power of *Janguisism* [sic], that it may well be doubted if *Simon Magus*, with all his sorceries, ever performed more surprising feats. They tell any person his thoughts, cause the branch of a tree to blossom and bear fruit within an hour, hatch an egg in their bosom in less than fifteen minutes, producing whatever bird may be demanded, and make it fly about the room, and execute many other prodigies that need not be enumerated.[19]

Here we see a conflation of several different groups under the general label of "Jaugi" or "Fakire." They include assorted types of ascetics, some certainly belonging to a variety of Śaiva traditions, others perhaps being Vaiṣṇavas. They include in all likelihood both genuine practitioners as well as those posing as such as a means of obtaining alms. Later in the account, which Bernier highlights as describing something "totally different," we also see alchemical specialists who are, for our purposes, to be distinguished from the concurrently mentioned street magicians who demonstrate seemingly superhuman powers purely for entertainment.[20]

Of note here is the variety of models that could be reasonably recognizable as Yogis. Over the next three centuries, these "faces" of the Yogi—in particular, the ascetic, the mystic, and the magician—would continue to emerge, converge, and diverge in the Western imagination. It should be noted that, as White has argued, the Westerners who originally encountered and therefore reported upon Yogis were not only outsiders but, by virtue of this fact, were likely to experience these encounters in public places such as markets, temples, and pilgrimage sites. They were consequently exposed to very specific kinds of Yogis who might have been expected to congregate around such locations.[21] The Yogi's public relations, at least as far as the first three centuries of his exposure to the West are concerned, are thus characterized by two converging phenomena: the tendency of publicly visible Yogis to behave in shocking, ostentatious, and sometimes unscrupulous ways as a matter of livelihood, and the desire of Western audiences for the shocking, the exotic, and the possibly magical. It is then no surprise that Yogi ascetics and magicians occupied more than their share of the limelight through the end of the nineteenth century. It is largely only with the arrival of self-proclaimed

Yogis, such as Vivekananda and his successors, that American audiences began to recognize the flavor of meditative mystics that had historically been associated with a much less socially visible kind of practice. Nevertheless, most human Yogis who achieved any kind of success in attracting American audiences would ultimately come to embody all three faces, at least to some extent and at times in spite of themselves.

Yogi Ascetics

Gratuitous descriptions of the Yogi's various ascetic acts, such as seen in Bernier's account, are a generally uniform feature of the travel account genre where India is concerned. Such accounts translate with great consistency—no doubt in large part because the sources routinely plagiarize their predecessors rather than gathering any additional ethnographic data—into late nineteenth- and early twentieth-century European and American texts, both scholarly and popular.

Of course, textual sources were not the sole source of such Western impressions. Photographs of Indian ascetics were wildly popular during the colonial era. As with the verbal accounts, they were clearly crafted to invoke a kind of morbid fascination—a voyeuristic indulgence not unlike the allure of the freak show— that focused on the ascetic Yogi's various mortifications. Earlier travel accounts and colonial news media often included sketches, but with the popularization of photography in the mid-nineteenth century Yogis came to life for Western audiences in an entirely new way. Commercial photographic studios began to churn out volumes of photographs of foreign lands and peoples for the exoticism-hungry eyes of British consumers.

With the introduction of the carte-de-visite format (a small photo print roughly the size of a modern business card) in 1854, collectible images of Yogi portraits became particularly popular.[22] Individuals, who may or may not have been actual ascetics, would appear posed against increasingly elaborate (but almost always artificial) backdrops with a wide variety of props. By the twentieth century, the ascetic Yogi reclining on his bed of nails would become a universally recognizable image across Western books, newsprint, photographs, and postcards.[23] A 1913 *National Geographic* article entitled, "Religious Penances and Punishments Self-Inflicted by Hindu Holy Men" featured a particularly extensive photographic representation of the various austerities undertaken by such figures (see fig. 1.1).

This anthropological exposé arrived on the heels of Oman's pseudo-ethnographic account of India's ascetics in 1903. In addition to its extensive description of the identities and activities of India's many ascetic groups, along

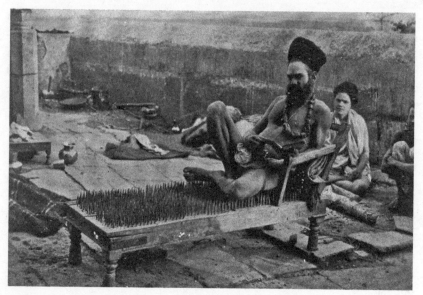

FIGURE 1.1 "Bed of Thorns," *National Geographic* 24 (1913)

with a collection of plates offering visual depictions of the same, Oman's work attempts to situate these individuals in their cultural context to the best of its author's ability. Interestingly, Oman, more so than any other Western interpreter of Yogis and their austerities, seeks to provide a rationale to make sense of these activities beyond citing deluded belief in their salvific effects:

> But the value of austerities for the attainment of practical ends, commendable or the reverse, and the power for good or evil possessed by the ascetic, are the considerations connected with asceticism which are most deeply graven on the Indian mind; and this fact enables us to appreciate the standpoint from which the Hindu looks up to the *sadhu* who has practiced, or may pretend to have practiced, austerities, as one who might help him to gain his ends, or, on the other hand, might hurl a curse at him with the most direful consequences.[24]

In short, the Yogi's practice of austerities, which captivate the Western imagination with their surface shock factor, is embroiled in a much larger system of power. These associations are obvious if one looks at the traditional role of Yogis in South Asian popular lore and religious systems of practice, but such ideological linkages do not always successfully translate into Western interpretations. In trying to represent the logic of the "Indian mind," Oman stumbles upon a millennia-old association between the metaphysical power of *tapas*, or ascetic practice, and superpower. His explanation is one of the few instances we find of a Western acknowledgment of this causal relationship between asceticism and the phenomenon that constitutes the public face of superpower: magic.

Generally speaking, if Western audiences had any notion of a causal association between asceticism and superpower, the direction of the relationship would likely have been reversed. That is, the Yogi is able to comfortably recline on his bed of nails or withstand any other such torturous activity because he is already in possession of some superhuman talent. If any such reason is cited for the Yogi's engagement in these activities, it is that they are displays of his powers of (in this case, self-)hypnotism. More often than not, however, the issue of superpower or magic is left out of the discussion of Yogic asceticism altogether. Yogis, it seems, are just simply gluttons for punishment. Consequently, the Yogi's identity as ascetic is increasingly separated from his identity as magician, though certain images—the bed of nails being a prime example—bridge the gap in the theatricality of both.

Yogi Magicians

The Yogi's various talents do occasionally manifest as a coherent identity. For instance, if one were to refer to the 1916 edition of the *Encyclopoedia of Religion and Ethics*, one would learn that

> the caste which is particularly devoted to magic as a vocation is that of the Yogīs, which is primarily Hindu but has Mohammadan elements affiliated to it. The Yogī claims to hold the material world in fee by the magical powers which he has acquired through the performance of religious austerities, but this claim soon degenerates into superstition of the worst type, and the Yogī in reality is little better than a common swindler, posing as a *faqīr*. . . . The Yogīs in particular claim power to transmute base metals into silver and gold—a claim which enables them (and those who personate them) to reap a great harvest from the credulous.[25]

Here we see the Yogi's asceticism and superhuman powers causally coupled in a bid for nothing short of world domination. However, such aspirations—aptly signified by the Yogi's pretensions to alchemy—are only swindlers' tricks. The Western public's fascination with what the Yogi could do, or at least what he could appear to do, often held an even stronger allure than the grotesquerie of his penances. Stories of Indian jugglers—the preferred term for such individuals, which in its older usage was a synonym for the magician but came conveniently close to being a homonym for the colloquial pronunciations of Yogi (*jogi*)—captivated an audience for whom the Orient was still alive with the kind of mystery that was no longer possible in the post-Enlightenment West.

Although early accounts ran a good chance of being met with fear of magic and witchcraft, Victorians came to pride themselves on their rationality and lack of superstition while simultaneously being fascinated with the possibility of the era's evolving metaphysical assumptions. For instance, in 1832 stories of Sheshal, a Madras brahmin better known as the "man that sat in the air," caused a flurry in the British press and were hailed as "some wonderful discovery in magnetism" before being debunked by the discovery of a steel support that held up the apparently levitating man.[26] Levitation, riding high on the vapors of Spiritualism, was always a popular phenomenon. Other time-proven staples included the mango trick—a version of which is described in Bernier's account—which usually involved a mango seed flourishing into a tree and even bearing fruit before the eyes of the observer. Snake-charming and live burial were also strong favorites.

Unlike the Yogi ascetics, who for most Westerners appeared only as distant "natives" accessible via narrative or, at best, photographic media, Yogi magicians brought the Orient alive on Western stages.[27] Though often billed as "fakirs," they frequently appeared dressed in elaborate robes and turbans, bedecked with jewels and feathers to play up the allure of Oriental luxe. Generally speaking, most of these men were actually Westerners who donned what they believed to be Oriental garb for effect. For instance, one Fakir of Ava, whose legal identity was Isaiah Harris Hughes from Essex, billed himself as "Chief of Staff of Conjurers to His Sublime Greatness the Nanka of Aristophae" and promised to "appear in his native costume, and will perform the most Astonishing Miracles of the East!" After a brief and unsuccessful stint in the American West during the mid-nineteenth century, the Fakir of Ava traded his robes for European formal wear and set off to thus perform in Australia.[28] Even the famous Charles Dickens once appeared as The Unparalleled Necromancer Rhia Rhama Rhoos at a charity event in 1849. It should be noted that both of these men wore exotic robes and brownface but performed tricks that were not in any particular way "Indian."[29] In this sense, the persona of an Oriental Yogi could be used to add a bit of spice to an otherwise lackluster stage performance. There were, of course, some actual South Asians, Middle Easterners, and Northern Africans (the Orient and its people were both rather ambiguous categories, after all) who made the best of their racial nonconformity by taking on such performative personae. However, they were arguably not only in the minority but were inserting themselves into a co-opted aesthetic that had initially been developed by their white counterparts at their expense.

Moreover, while Euro-American stage magicians were only all too glad to make use of Oriental costuming and even "Indian-inspired" illusions, they were careful to maintain that no actual magic was involved. Having already engaged in a longtime feud with the Spiritualists, who claimed metaphysical origins for their phenomena of levitation and even apparition, the professional illusionists were eager to show that similarly fantastic acts could be accomplished without any recourse to supernatural means. Yogi magicians—or more specifically stories of them—had a particular knack for inspiring a tendency toward credulity in Western audiences who longed to believe in the wonders of the Orient. This led to a kind of stage magic one-upmanship, as popular magicians such as John Nevil Maskelyne, Charles Bertram, and the famous Harry Houdini spent the better half of the century's turn debunking tales of Yogi magic by publicizing the techniques through which such feats could be accomplished. Maskelyne was particularly zealous on this point and in 1914 founded the Occult Committee, which, rather than devoting itself to the exploration of the supernatural as its name would suggest, was instead devoted entirely to disproving the legitimacy of such phenomena. Of special concern to the committee was proving the impossibility of a particular "Indian" phenomenon involving a free-floating rope.[30]

As Indian magic went, most paradigmatic of all was undoubtedly the Indian rope trick, which incorporated levitation into a live-action performance and by the twentieth century had become nearly as reminiscent of the Yogi as his bed of nails. In the "traditional" version of this trick, the Yogi or fakir would telekinetically raise a rope into the air and a young boy serving as his assistant would climb it, eventually disappearing from view. The magician would attempt to call back his assistant and, when the boy did not respond, would become angry and follow the boy up the rope, wielding a large knife. The magician would likewise disappear and moments later body parts, presumably belonging to the boy, would tumble to the ground. The magician would then climb down the rope, place the dismembered parts into a basket, out of which the boy would reappear unharmed. This illusion became particularly popular in stage magic and many versions—most of them far less elaborate—would be performed across Europe and America. The origins of the Indian rope trick would come to be traced by some to no lesser text than the philosopher Śaṃkara's ninth-century commentary on the *Vedānta Sūtra*.[31] However, historian Peter Lamont has argued that the illusion (which has never been successfully performed in its full form under open-air conditions) originated from a wildly popular but ultimately fictional news article that first appeared in the *Chicago Tribune* on August 8, 1890.

The article, entitled "It Is Only Hypnotism. How Indian Fakirs Deceive Those Who Watch Them," was in fact a spectacular example of Western attempts to naturalize the Yogi's powers. As the story went, Fred S. Ellmore, a Yale graduate with an interest in photography, along with his artist friend George Lessing had recently returned from India where they had seen a street fakir perform several extraordinary feats. The performance culminated in a basic version of the then-novel rope trick in which the fakir threw a ball of twine into the air that subsequently disappeared from sight, a boy climbed the twine and disappeared roughly forty feet from the ground, and the twine itself disappeared a moment later. Ellmore and Lessing were both prepared for and skeptical of such wonders and so, while Lessing sketched the progression of the act, Ellmore took photographs of the same. The photographs, in contrast to the sketches, revealed no twine, no boy, but only the fakir sitting on the ground. As the article glibly explained, "Mr Fakir has simply hypnotized the entire crowd, but he couldn't hypnotize the camera."[32] As Lamont reveals, the entire story was a hoax penned by one John Elbert Wilkie, and a retraction was printed in the *Chicago Tribune* four months later—but by then the story had been reprinted multiple times and translated into nearly every European language.[33] Not only was the retraction generally ignored by the public, but the hypnotism-based debunking offered by the fictional authors also gradually fell by the wayside. The performance of the Indian rope trick became a holy grail for those seeking to discover the wonders of India.

Ultimately we can take away two very important points from the story of the Indian rope trick. One is the enormous cultural power of tropes and narratives to influence and even shape reality. The other point concerns the underlying origins of the Yogi's superpowers. Those who wanted to believe were much more able to do so if they were able to ascribe the Yogi's seemingly magical abilities to the powers of the mind, and more specifically to the powers of hypnotism, whether the Yogi was thought to apply such powers to himself or to others. Even the most ardent skeptics could often be found attempting to explain the otherwise unexplainable claiming that the Yogi used hypnotism, in the case of seemingly supernatural occurrences, or that he had relied on the sheer force of his personal charm, in cases of the remarkable sway that he seemed to have over the finances of the social elite.

Yogi Mystics

It is important to emphasize that when Vivekananda stepped onto the stage of the World Parliament of Religions in 1893, he did so neither as a ragged ascetic nor as a bejeweled magician. Of course, whether he was at the time presenting himself as a Yogi per se is also up for debate. Nevertheless, Vivekananda, at that moment or during the American tour that followed would hardly have been comprehensible to his audiences had they not already been exposed to a very different kind of Yogi.

Although most histories of Hinduism—what to say of yoga—in America will begin flourishingly with Vivekananda, some do include a brief preamble concerning the Transcendentalists, namely Ralph Waldo Emerson and Henry David Thoreau.[34] Emerson, as journal entries made in his younger days will attest, initially appeared quite perturbed by the "Yoguees of Hindostan" and "their extravagancies and practices of self torture"[35] though he later came to admire a good number of Indian texts. However, while Emerson's interest in India and its religious literature was rather diffuse, Thoreau expressed a rather targeted interest in Yogis, even going so far as to identify with what he believed to be their ideologies. Of course, while the rest of America was busy absorbing missionary accounts of widow burnings and frightful ascetics, Thoreau was sojourning at Walden Pond and reading the *Bhagavad Gītā*. Thus, his notion of what it might have meant to be a Yogi was perhaps rather different from the perspectives of many of his contemporaries.

Whereas the chief manifestation of Indian ideology in Emerson's work appears as a kind of spiritual aesthetics, Thoreau had a more utilitarian approach. He read the texts available to him as instruction manuals. While at Walden, he appears to have tried his hand—or rather his head—at meditation, though to unclear degrees of success. In an 1849 letter to Harrison Gray Otis Blake, Thoreau writes:

> Depend upon it that, rude and careless as I am, I would fain practice the *yoga* faithfully. . . . "The yogi, absorbed in contemplation, contributes in his degree to creation: he breathes a divine perfume, he hears wonderful things. Divine forms traverse him without tearing him, and, united to the nature which is proper to him, he goes, he acts as animating original matter." To some extent, and at rare intervals even I am a yogin.[36]

The incorporated quotation, which Thoreau drew from a translation of the *Harivaṃśa*, was a favorite of his.[37] To what extent Thoreau experienced such visions and felt himself to be "animating original matter" remains ambiguous, but such passages make it clear that he did make a genuine attempt to take his practice beyond simple aesthetic contemplation. Thus, as Stefanie Syman has argued, we can perhaps legitimately say that "Thoreau was a Yogi, in part, because he tried to be one."[38] Insomuch as Thoreau's stance reflects a universalization of yogic practice—oftentimes requiring a break with traditional lineage-based modes of transmission and an ongoing transformation of ritual practice—he is certainly among the first data points in a powerful trajectory of how yoga and Yogis have been defined.

When Moncure Conway, Thoreau's friend and admirer, eulogized him in 1866 as something like a Yogi, the old language of asceticism began to take on rather new meanings. Referring to Thoreau's time at Walden, Conway wrote:

Like the pious Yógi of the East one, so long motionless whilst gazing on
the sun that knotty plants encircled his neck and the cast snake-skin his
loins, and the birds built their nests upon his shoulders, this seer and natu-
ralist seemed by equal consecration to have become a part of the field and
forest amid which he dwelt.[39]

The imagery is striking in its subtle differences from earlier accounts of Yogi figures. No mention is made of the Yogi's emaciated limbs, filthy skin, or the nails
that grow so long from neglect that they come to hang down or even pierce his
skin, though one can certainly imagine that all of these conditions must be present if the plants have had time to accommodate him in their growth patterns.
Instead, the Yogi becomes literally one with nature, which carries an altogether
different connotation from the "unnatural" neglect of their bodies undertaken by
the ascetics of other accounts. Through this shift in focus, Thoreau becomes the
first symbol of a Yogi who, ragged as he may be, symbolizes something other than
ignorant superstition. In turn, by being absorbed into the discourse of a nature-
oriented Romanticism, the Yogi becomes more comprehensible to cultural elites
for whom this ideology holds capital. It is important to note that while the "mystical Orient" was in many ways still a characterization that was used to devalue
Indian culture by painting it as passive, introverted, and ultimately irrational,[40] it
also proved to be a powerful point of attraction to those for whom mysticism did
not hold such negative valences.

Even more influential, however, was Edwin Arnold's *Light of Asia*, which
brought Indian religion to a far broader audience and colored the way in which
Westerners saw Asia for decades to come. First published in 1876 but ultimately
going through over a hundred editions in England and America, the text was
a novella-length narrative poem recounting the life of the historical Buddha.
Highly sympathetic, the account depicted him as almost Christ-like in his
purity and enlightenment.[41] This was the first exposure that many Westerners
would have had to Buddhism of any kind, but it is crucial to note that this was
an Indian Buddhism and thus Arnold's narrative employed many of the tropes
that Westerns audiences would have recognized from depictions of India in
general. Among these was an account of the familiarly grotesque Yogi ascetics,
whose ways the Buddha comes to reject as not only overly extreme but ultimately
deluded:

> *Midway on Ratnagiru's groves of calm,*
> *Beyond the city, below the caves,*
> *Lodged such as hold the body foe to soul,*
> *And flesh a beast which men must chain and tame*

With bitter pains, till sense of pain is killed,
And tortured nerves vex torturer no more—
Yogis and Brahmacharis, Bhikshus, all
A gaunt and mournful band, dwelling apart.
Some day and night had stood with lifted arms
Till—drained of blood and withered by disease—
Their slowly-wasting joints and stiffened limbs
Jutted from sapless shoulders like dead forks
From forest trunks. Others had clenched their hands
So long with so fierce a fortitude,
The claw-like nails grew through the festered palm.
Some walked on sandals spiked; some with sharp flints
Gashed breast and brow and thigh, scarred these with fire,
Threaded their flesh with jungle thorns and spits,
Besmeared with mud and ashes, crouching foul
In rags of dead men wrapped about their loins.
Certain there were inhabited the spots
Where death pyres smouldered, cowering defiled
With corpses for their company, and kites
Screaming around them o'er the funeral-spoils;
Certain who cried five hundred times a day
The names of Shiva, wound with darting snakes
About their sun-tanned necks and hollow flanks,
One palsied foot drawn up against the ham.
So gathered they, a grievous company;
Crowns blistered by the blazing heat, eyes bleared,
Sinews and muscles shrivelled, visages
Haggard and wan as slain men's, five days dead;
Here crouched one in the dust who noon by noon
Meted a thousand grains of millet out,
Ate it with famished patience, seed by seed,
And so starved on; there one who bruised his pulse
With bitter leaves lest palate should be pleased;
And next, a miserable saint self-maimed,
Eyeless and tongueless, sexless, crippled, deaf;
The body by the mind being thus stripped
For glory of much suffering, and the bliss
Which they shall win—say holy books—whose woe
Shames gods that send us woe, and makes men gods
Stronger to suffer than hell is to harm.[42]

Against the disfigured and self-destructive Yogis, Arnold represents the Buddha in formidable contrast. Having regained his strength and vigor after leaving excessive austerities behind, he is described as "Sitting serene, with perfect virtue walled / As is a stronghold by its gates and ramps."[43] Thus, despite the potential strangeness of the Buddha's concomitant metaphysical doctrines—for which Arnold expresses an admiration but ultimately devalues in the face of Christianity's superiority—the public was presented with a new and far more appealing model of Indian mysticism. It is important to note that the Buddha was not a "Yogi," nor was he a "Hindu," and thus it would be tempting to dismiss his impact on the formation of the former persona. However, given the general lack of differentiation when it came to all things Oriental in the mind of the contemporary American public, the general image would have been understood simply as that of a "Mystic from the East." And it proved to be a memorable image.

This alternate model of Yogihood would slowly pick up steam as Western interest in Indian thought became more earnest. The Yogi ascetics and magicians would always be a passing curiosity, but in the Yogi mystic Americans and other Westerners increasingly recognized a truth that some felt to be missing from their own religions. A brief mention should be made in this context of Theosophy and its Mahatmas, especially insofar as some of them were in fact declared to be Indian Yogis. However, the Mahatmas were more ideas than they were people, and as such they will be discussed more fully in the following chapter. As far as people were concerned, the Indian intellectual elites' acceptance of such figures as universal adepts was reflective of an ideological shift that had much to do with the neo-Hindu reforms of organizations such as the Brahmo Samāj, whose religious leanings had strong universalistic tendencies.

Indians themselves, largely emboldened by Western affection for texts such as the *Yoga Sūtras*, which were thought to represent a philosophical, meditative, and therefore pure yoga, were seeking to reformulate the understanding of what constituted authentic yogic practice. This caused the would-be ethnographer Oman to observe in 1889:

> Happily, there are already signs which indicate that even such educated natives as cannot emancipate themselves from a belief in *yoga-vidya*—national beliefs die hard—are beginning to be ashamed of the dirty, indolent, and repulsive mendicants who perambulate the country, and, for the credit of the so-called yog science, pretend that the *real* yogis are very different from these unclean and disgusting objects of popular veneration.
>
> With the spread of Western ideas, and with the growth of new objects of ambition created by intimate contact with the restless civilization and

free institutions of Europe, the yogi and his system will necessarily occupy a diminishing place in the hearts of the people of India.[44]

Oman was right on one point. The roaming Yogis were by now seen as a national embarrassment by Westernized Indian intellectual elites as they, like the caste system and widow burning, represented everything that was hopelessly backward about Indian civilization. However, rather than edging the Yogi out altogether, this forward march of civilization yielded still new kinds of Yogis who could be viewed as sources of national, and even more importantly Hindu, pride rather than disgrace.

Vivekananda surely had a monumental hand in this phenomenon. At the time of Oman's assertion, Vivekananda was still struggling to rebuild a community following the death of his guru, Ramakrishna. He and his associates, however, were part of an increasingly nationalistic neo-Hindu reform movement that would seek to reclaim Hinduism's place of honor on the world stage. By 1903 in America, one Yogi Ramacharaka—also known as New Thought author William Walker Atkinson—has the following to say of his Indian namesakes:

> The Western student is apt to be somewhat confused in his ideas regarding the Yogis and their philosophy and practice. Travelers to India have written great tales about the hordes of fakirs, mendicants and mountebanks who infest the great roads of India and the streets of its cities, and who impudently claim the title "Yogi." The Western student is scarcely to be blamed for thinking of the typical Yogi as an emaciated, fanatical, dirty, ignorant Hindu, who either sits in a fixed posture until his body becomes ossified, or else holds his arm up in the air until it becomes stiff and withered and forever after remains in that position, or perhaps clenches his fist and holds it tight until his fingernails grow through the palms of his hands. That these people exist is true, but their claim to the title "Yogi" seems as absurd to the true Yogi as does the claim to the title "Doctor" on the part of the man who pares one's corns seem to the eminent surgeon, or as does the title of "Professor," as assumed by the street corner vendor of worm medicine, seem to the President of Harvard or Yale.[45]

Atkinson, as far as history can attest, had no personal experience with either the "emaciated, fanatical, dirty, ignorant Hindu" or the "true" Yogi to whom he implicitly refers. At least not on Indian soil. This particular passage, however, appears in publication some ten years after Vivekananda first arrived in the United States. Given that much of the metaphysical framework that characterizes Atkinson's multitudinous body of publications appears to be lifted straight from

Vivekananda's *Raja Yoga* (1896), it would not strain the imagination that when Atkinson refers to true Yogis, he is referring quite pointedly to Vivekananda.

Vivekananda

It is important to note that Emerson actually thought the *Bhagavad Gītā* was a Buddhist text. Historically speaking, Yogis certainly need not be Hindu. However, Emerson's and the general American public's confusion had little to do with the historical lack of boundaries between different forms of Indian yogic practice and much more to do with the historical lack of knowledge about Asian religions in nineteenth-century America. Consequently, it is not surprising that Vivekananda was frequently referred to by the press as a "Buddhist priest," even following his lectures. This is likely attributable both to the popularity of Arnold's *Light of Asia* and to Vivekananda's own frequent allusions to the Buddha.[46] To bring the matter full circle, it is likely that Vivekananda's penchant for mentioning the Buddha stemmed from his own admiration of Arnold's text, to which he would occasionally allude, and it is even conceivable that Arnold's rendition of the Oriental sage had a formative effect on Vivekananda's public persona,[47] yielding a self-reinforcing image of the Yogi.

Vikekananda's childhood biography appears to be somewhat conflated with that of his guru, Ramakrishna. Vivekananda himself recounted to Margaret Noble, who would eventually become Sister Nivedita, that he had begun practicing meditation at the age of seven and had successfully attained *samādhi* by eight.[48] However, Vivekananda's participation in the Brahmo Samāj appears to have been prompted more by seeking a venue for his musical expertise than any intense spiritual thirst, or even interest in the message of social reform as he himself claimed. Vivekananda, who was then Narendra Nath Datta, fancied himself an intellectual, and was originally skeptical of the illiterate mystic Ramakrishna, who would later become his guru. The mystic, on the other hand, was utterly enchanted with the talented youth.[49] After the untimely death of Vivekananda's father, Ramakrishna, having survived not one but two similar losses with the passing of his father and elder brother, must have been a source of significant psychological support. However, even accounting for the close emotional bond, it is questionable how much Vivekananda would have gleaned from his teacher in the realm of yogic practice. Before his father's death in 1884, Vivekananda's visits to Ramakrishna's community at Dakshineshwar were very irregular, and afterwards financial difficulties within the family consumed much of his time.

Vivekananda's spiritual exercises, as far as can be ascertained, involved basic meditation. When Ramakrishna fell ill shortly after the intensification of their relationship, Vivekananda began spending more time at the compound and practicing various austerities. He would smear himself with ashes and don the garb of a renunciant. Incidentally, he would later blame his diabetes on this period of asceticism. After Ramakrishna's passing in 1886, much of the patronage for his Cassipore establishment dwindled. Vivekananda and his fellow young aspirants were reluctant to let go of the property and dreamed of erecting a temple there to honor their guru. The group, now largely estranged from Ramakrishna's householder disciples, established a sort of bohemian commune where they would go naked, share communal meals from food that they begged in the streets, and smoke hookah while discussing Vedāntin scriptures. However, given the strained financial situation, Vivekananda's austerities were as much compulsory as they might have been voluntary.[50]

Of special interest, given the current topic, is the relatively short amount of time that Vivekananda spent with Ramakrishna and the apparently spiritually therapeutic rather than instructive nature of their relationship. Even more important, Elizabeth De Michelis asserts that, based on the available evidence, one thing is certain:

> Ramakrishna never formally initiated the future Vivekananda and the other young devotees. This is a stark fact that both Vivekananda and the early Ramakrishna movement have been at pains to underplay and to counterbalance with informal or "mystical" types of initiation.[51]

Thus, whatever his relationship with Ramakrishna may have been, to the extent that Vivekananda was a Yogi he was certainly a self-made one, who was to no small extent influenced by Western and Westernized models of what such an identity entailed. This fact would also have profound ramifications with regard to the kind of practice that Vivekananda might have taught while in America. Ramakrishna's own spiritual practice was complex and eclectic. Although it was overall ecstatic and devotional in character, he did receive significant instruction from a female tantric guru known as Bhairavi Brahmani. It does not appear, however, that he transmitted any brand of systematized tantric *sādhana* to Vivekananda.

Nor was Vivekananda a proponent of the then emerging modern reincarnation of *āsana*-based (postural) *haṭha* yoga. Vivekananda suffered from diabetes (possibly genetic in nature) from his teenage years onward, and this, coupled with his sedentary lifestyle and unhealthy personal habits including diet and predilections toward smoking and snuff, led to a host of other ailments. It is attested that during his Indian travels in 1890 he had contact with a famous ascetic and mystic named Pavhari Baba at Ghazipur, from whom he attempted to learn *haṭha* yoga. However, Vivekananda quickly abandoned the enterprise due to its difficulty, owing to the intense physical exercise and strict dietary regimen required by the program.[52] Consequently, though we do have reports of Vivekananda giving practical lessons in the United States,[53] these, in keeping with the character of his published *Raja Yoga*, would have been largely theoretical in nature and emphasized basic breathing exercises and meditation techniques.

Vivekananda's less-than-ideal fitness did not, however, seem to detract from his imposing appearance in the eyes of his American admirers. Cornelius Johannes Heijblom, a Dutch immigrant who would go on to become Swami Atulananda, saw Vivekananda in New York in 1899, about which he reminisced:

> What a giant, what strength, what manliness, what a personality! Everyone near him looks so insignificant in comparison. . . . What was it that gave Swamiji his distinction? Was it his height? No, there were gentlemen there taller than he was. Was it his build? No, there were near him some very fine specimens of American manhood. It seemed to be more in the expression of the face than anything else. Was it his purity? What was it? . . .
> I remember what had been said of Lord Buddha—"a lion amongst men."[54]

It is beyond doubt that much in such impressions is owed to Vivekananda's immense personal presence and charisma. Josephine MacLeod, who would become an ardent admirer, described him in 1895 as "the fiery missionary whose physique was like a wrestler's and whose eyes were deep black."[55] Transfixed, she further recalls: "I saw with these very eyes . . . Krishna himself standing there and preaching the Gita. That was my first wonderful vision. I stared and stared . . . I saw only the figure and all else vanished."[56] Such allusions to the Buddha and Krishna are telling in that they signify figures who would have been familiar to an audience of this time as models of Indian spirituality in its "purest" form. Both of these figures, furthermore, might have been associated with something that Americans were beginning to recognize as yoga—Krishna explicitly in his teachings in the *Bhagavad Gītā*, the Buddha more implicitly through his meditative character—but neither of them was anything like the popularly familiar Yogis of the time.

However, the impressions left by Vivekananda had as much, or perhaps more, to do with his presence than with the content of his lectures. Martha Brown Fincke, who saw Vivekananda lecture in the college town of Northampton, writes:

> The name of India was familiar to me from my earliest childhood. Had not my mother almost decided to marry a young man who went as a missionary to India, and did not a box from our Church Missionary Association

go each year to Zenanas? India was a hot land where snakes abounded and "the heathen in his blindness bows down to wood and stone." It is astonishing how little an eager reader like myself knew about the history or literature of that great country. . . . To talk with a real Indian would be a chance indeed. . . . Of the lecture that evening I can recall nothing. The imposing figure on the platform in red robe, orange cord, and yellow turban, I do remember and the wonderful mastery of the English language with its rich sonorous tones, but the ideas did not take root in my mind or else the many years since then have obliterated them.[57]

What Fincke does remember was the symposium that followed, in which Vivekananda faced down a "row of black-coated and somewhat austere gentlemen" who, with their volleys of biblical references and philosophical allusions, argued for the superiority of Christianity. To this onslaught, Vivekananda replied with his own quotes from the same, leaving Finke wondering:

Why were my sympathies not with those of my own world? Why did I exult in the air of freedom that blew through the room as the Swami broadened the scope of Religion till it embraced all mankind? Was it that his words found an echo in my own longings, or was it simply the magic of his personality? I cannot tell, I only know that I felt triumphant with him.[58]

Fincke's account does hint at one ideological tactic that was crucial to Vivekananda's appeal: his universalism. However, the majority of her memories are nevertheless dominated by physical and emotional impressions. Other observers were even more direct about the extent to which Vivekananda's presence overwhelmed the content of his discourse. One older English woman, for instance, observed: "I love the Swami talk . . . I can't understand much of the philosophy but his voice and gestures charm me. I seem to be seeing someone out of the Bible."[59] Another woman was simply "fascinated by his turban."[60]

Vivekananda himself was not oblivious to the fetishism with which he was often treated. He wrote to a friend in India in 1894: "Just now I am living as the guest of an old lady in a village near Boston. . . . I have an advantage in living with her . . . and she has the advantage of inviting her friends over here and showing them a curio from India."[61] He clearly understood the extent to which he was indebted to the American women—and they were overwhelmingly women—who patronized him, and he made frequent moves both publicly and in letters to praise them for their virtue, education, and spirituality. At times, however, his façade would break, which happened all the more often after he returned to India.

At these moments, he would assert that the same women were "not steady, serious, or sincere." In Boston, especially, "the women are all faddists, all fickle, merely bent on following something new and strange."[62]

Aside from being treated as a novelty item, Vivekananda also came up against the expectations that American audiences had of Yogis. "Give Us Some Miracles!" demanded the Detroit *Evening News* when Vivekananda turned out to have little more than philosophy up his sleeve. It was deemed by the public that he should "put up or shut up."[63] Vivekananda, in turn, not only had little flair for the supernatural but was fundamentally ambivalent about his role in the West. Contrary to the popular belief among his American followers, he revealed a rather practical rationalization for his presence on the Western stage. He viewed his journey to America above all as a financial venture aimed at raising funds to elevate the condition of his home nation, summarizing the matter as follows: "As our country is poor in social virtues, so this country is lacking in spirituality. I give them spirituality and they give me money."[64] This statement appeared in a private correspondence and was issued before Vivekananda actually arrived on American shores. However, it seems that time spent with his American disciples did little to abate his ambivalence as a spiritual teacher to the West. Toward the end of his American sojourn, he declared to an inquiring woman in San Francisco: "Madam, I am not teaching religion. I am selling my own brain for money to help my people."[65]

Nor was every person Vivekananda encountered entirely convinced of his spiritual credentials. Certain Christian Scientists, for instance, responded somewhat skeptically. Ashton Jonson, enthusiastic over his sermons but shocked to see a Yogi in a state of such bodily ill health, wrote to Sarah Bull:

> I no more condemn or criticize him than I do a child who falls down and hurts itself. If I am asked to recognize that Swami is manifesting the highest Divine consciousness in this disease . . . I do not feel that the highest consciousness can ever demand a diseased body in which to manifest. Of course I do not pretend to worship Swami's feet as Miss Noble does.[66]

That Vivekananda was not able to appear coherent as a Yogi to Jonson had as much to do with the extent to which Yogis, by way of the Theosophical Mahatmas, had been incorporated into the American metaphysical worldview as with Vivekananda's own ambivalent Yogihood.

Although Vivekananda became increasingly absorbed and indeed invested in mysticism as his health worsened, it is not at all clear that he had ever meant to present himself as a self-realized adept for any reason other than gaining credibility with his American benefactors. His grasp on this persona was historically rather tenuous, as the more disaffected of his public and private statements illustrate. Furthermore, some of the attacks against Vivekananda originated from what should have been his own camp. For example, Pratap Chandra Mazumdar, who represented the Brahmo Samāj at the World Parliament of Religions, accused Vivekananda of being a "Bohemian impostor who preached a pseudo-Hinduism."[67] Thus Vivekananda was never quite at home in—and never quite conformed to the ideals of—either the American metaphysical community or the heart of the nationalism neo-Hindu movement, two groups who have since made him their model representative.

Early American Yogis

Despite his extraordinarily long shadow, Vivekananda was actually a rather minor presence on the landscape of American Yogis. He arrived in 1893 and toured the United States (with two brief visits to England) until 1897. He returned to America and Europe between 1899 and 1902 and established a handful of Vedanta Society centers, but his declining health reduced his visibility. His longtime associate, Swami Abhedananda, did however join him in England in 1896 and went on to continue Vivekananda's work in New York. Abhedananda remained in the United States for the better part of twenty-five years, finally departing back to India in 1921.

During his time in New York, Abhedananda maintained an active Vedanta Society center where he reputedly taught basic postural *haṭha* yoga and meditation.[68] His *How to Be a Yogi* (1902) affirms the historical and religious universality of yoga and advocates a "practical spirituality." Likely having picked up on his audience's concerns with health, Abhedananda declares that the goal of *haṭha* yoga is "the cure of disease through breathing exercises and the regulation of diet and of the general habits of daily life."[69] Notably, right alongside this claim, rests his assertion that a Yogi "can fascinate or madden another by his optical powers. . . . A Yogi can likewise read the thoughts of another by looking at his eyes; for according to the Yogi the eye is the index of the mind."[70] Of course, Abhedananda's audience would not have been shocked to learn that hypnotism was within the purview of a Yogi's powers. However, he is careful to note not only that "the process of hypnotism or mesmerism verifies this claim" but that Yogis "do not get [these powers] from outside. These powers are dormant in every individual, and through practice the Yogis bring them out."[71] In this way, Abhedananda continued Vivekananda's project of universalizing yoga and, with it, the Yogi. He emphasized that the Yogi is not in fact akin to the "fakir" or "juggler"—associations for which he blames the Theosophists—but rather to the "Rishis" or "Seers of Truth." Thus, as in many of Vivekananda's writings, which we

will examine in the next chapter, we see a denunciation of Yogis as unsavory characters practicing black magic while at the same time certain superhuman powers
are affirmed through an appeal to the universal power of the mind.

Some Yogis, like Vivekananda, came to the United States for the specific purpose of giving lectures or demonstrations and quickly departed back to India.
Shri Yogendra, for instance, can be credited with some of the first *āsana* demonstrations in the United States in the early 1920s.[72] Overall, Vivekananda's success
brought a number of Indian intellectuals, Yogi types and otherwise, to America's
universities and the communities surrounding them. Some came with the goal of
attaining degrees, others simply to engage in intellectual exchange. Most of these,
however, were temporary visitors rather than permanent settlers.

In addition to the swamis associated with the Vedanta Society and other visitors, a number of more "professional" Yogis slowly trickled in during the first
few decades of the twentieth century. The first wave of South Asian immigrants
arrived chiefly between 1907 and 1924. The Immigration Act of 1917, also known
as the "Asiatic Barred Zone Act," effectively added Indians to the growing number
of Asian groups whose entry into the United States was barred alongside other
"undesirable" categories of individuals. In 1923 a Supreme Court decision denying South Asians access to citizenship and the subsequent Immigration Act of
1924 reinforced these prohibitive laws. This first wave of immigrants came primarily from the Punjab, with small numbers originating in Oudh, Bengal, and
Gujarat, and consisted primarily of Sikhs and a small Muslim minority. More
precisely, Sikhs constituted approximately 85 to 90 percent of these early immigrants, Muslims accounted for another 10 percent, and actual Hindus (as distinct
from members of the aforementioned groups, which were popularly referred to as
"Hindus" once in the United States) were consequently quite rare.[73]

For many of these early South Asian immigrants, the desire to spread spiritual
knowledge was low on the list of considerations when choosing to leave their
homeland. Instead, they were part of a vast labor diaspora fleeing exploitative
colonial economic policies. A small minority were radical intellectuals who saw
themselves as political refugees in the face of repressive British rule.[74] Most of
the former group settled on the Pacific Coast, working on the Western Pacific
Railroad and in the lumber mills of Oregon and Washington. Because many were
agricultural workers, a large number also settled in or were driven down to the
Central Valley of California, where such labor was available and opportunities for
a small measure of social mobility were more plentiful. Some, primarily Bengali
Muslims, made their way into the American South, earning a living as traveling
"peddlers" who appealed to Americans' growing taste for the Oriental.[75] A few
men, however, some formally educated and some less so, were ingenious enough
to realize that the same aspects of their identity that made them so vulnerable

as targets of racism and ethnic exclusion could be transformed into a form of cultural capital.

A. K. Mozumdar arrived in Seattle from Calcutta in 1903 and set out to teach what was arguably the first form of "Christian Yoga" on the market. Mozumdar maintained a small following in Spokane for about sixteen years, lecturing to the community and working closely with the local branch of the Theosophical Society, New Thought group, and Unity Church, as well as publishing a regular periodical entitled *Christian Yoga Monthly*. After 1919, he relocated to Los Angeles, from where he launched himself onto a broader lecture circuit along the west coast and across the Midwest.[76]

Mozumdar was also the first individual of South Asian descent to be granted American citizenship in 1913, though it was later quite tragically revoked after the landmark case of *United States v. Bhagat Singh Thind* (<u>261 U.S. 204</u>), in 1923, which subsequently barred South Asians from citizenship until the passage of the Luce–Celler Act in 1946. However, though Thind would come to be remembered for this case, in which he valiantly tried and failed to contest the arbitrary nature of racial categorization, he also left a legacy as a spiritual author and teacher. Thind was a Punjabi Sikh who came to the United States in 1913 to pursue higher education, and he did indeed ultimately earn his doctorate from the University of California at Berkeley. He was deeply influenced by the Transcendentalists— especially Emerson, Whitman, and Thoreau—and wove their universalist spirituality together with Sikhism in his own teachings.

While some like Mozumdar and Thind focused their teachings on devotional and philosophical themes, others, such as Yogi Rishi Singh Gherwal, Yogi Wassan Singh, Yogi Hari Rama, and then-Swami Yogananda taught a more physically-oriented practice. As will be further discussed in chapter 4, though Gherwal was the only one to prescribe exercises that would today be recognizable as postural yoga, Yogananda, Hari Rama, and Yogi Wassan incorporated other forms of calisthenics with distinctively yogic goals. Such Yogis often struggled to meet the needs of audiences who were interchangeably looking for familiar images of ascetics, magicians, mystics, and sometimes all three at once. They followed a well-established lecture circuit, participated in vaudeville productions,[77] and published a number of philosophical and instructive volumes on yoga. Such publications varied vastly in both quality and originality.

For instance, Yogi Wassan's 1927 magnum opus, *Secrets of the Himalaya Mountain Masters and Ladder to Cosmic Consciousness*, features a vaguely *haṭha* yogic model, relying upon a system of plexuses opened along the principal energetic channels, which constitute "The Secret Key of Opana Yama" or "the System used by Householders to develop without excessive practice." A combination of diet, basic calisthenics, and specialized exercises promises to produce a "Super-Man" and "Super-Woman" endowed with perfect bodily health and telepathy, as well as the power of self-projection through an "ethereal body." The book is a rather dense volume, containing a multitude of *mantras* in corrupted Sanskrit and of indeterminate origin, lists of various stages of attainment, and instructions concerning various practices, some of which appear rather ill-advised as they require one to stare directly into the sun for lengthy periods of time. This is followed by a set of recipes, some of which are for bathing the eyes—unsurprising since most of the "Occult Concentration" exercises seem to involve some form of optic manipulation—while others are for homemade candy. The end lapses into practical miscellanea ranging from "How I make my Chicken Soup," to "What I Should Do if I Should Have a Hemorrhage or Diarrhea," to "How I Shampoo My Hair."[78]

A special mention should be made of Pierre Arnold Bernard, also known as the "Omnipotent Oom," who may very well deserve the title of America's first real domestic Yogi. Bernard's biography still remains a bit murky, but journalist Robert Love has recently done much to dispel at least a measure of the mystery. Bernard was born Perry Arnold Baker of Leon, Iowa, in 1876. This seems like an unlikely point of origin for a superstar Yogi, though perhaps not so much more unlikely than Lincoln, Nebraska, where, in 1889, young Perry met the teacher who would change his life. Bernard's guru was Sylvais Hamati, a Syrian Indian who had emigrated from Calcutta for reasons unknown. By the time he encountered Bernard, Hamati was making a reasonable living for himself as an itinerant tutor of "Vedic philosophy." It turned out, however, that Hamati was a veritable tantric Yogi and so initiated Bernard into an ancient lineage of practice. By 1896 Bernard and Hamati had relocated to San Francisco where Bernard, with a couple of invented degrees in tow, began marketing himself as a teacher of hypnotism, yoga, and other occult practices. His signature demonstration, which he called "Kali Mudra," involved entering into a deep trance while surgical needles were used to pierce various parts of his face. Bernard was ultimately able to place himself at the head of a circle of wealthy benefactors-cum-disciples, male and female, whom he organized into a secret society called the Tantrik Order after the fashion of the Freemasons and Theosophists.[79] Controversy and run-ins with the law forced Bernard to relocate a number of times, and he established several lodges of the Order across the Pacific Northwest before finally settling in New York.

Bernard's system of practice emphasized the sexual nature of tantric ritual—though to what extent the practices reflected any known Indian system is not clear—and he took on a series of female students as his sacred consorts or "nautch girls." In 1910 two of his close female disciples, Zelia Hopp and Gertrude Leo, facilitated his arrest, though perhaps not altogether intentionally, on the charges of kidnapping and false imprisonment. The media went into an immediate frenzy, though the case was ultimately dismissed and Bernard, together with his new partner Blanche De Vries, moved to Nyack where he would spend the rest of his days running what is perhaps best described as a yoga country club. As Bernard himself articulated it, his philosophy claimed:

> The purpose of human happiness is the purpose of Yoga, therefore what we are to understand by the Tantrik Order is simply that it is a body of men, Yogis, who for their evolution, for their happiness, follow a certain system, a certain science of Life, which being in accordance with nature is best suited to bring about the consummation which everybody desires, happiness.[80]

To this end, his disciples spent their days at the Clarkstown Country Club, according to the *Los Angeles Times* as "men and women, all garbed alike in black bloomers and white stockings, romping in the broad lawns or practicing strange exercises—exercises which appeared to be some weird, fantastic form of calisthenics."[81]

Finally, there were the Yogis who were not Yogis at all but simply adopted the persona for a variety of reasons. One such person was Yogi Ramacharaka, who never had a physical existence at all but was rather the nom-de-plume of the New Thought author William Walter Atkinson, created to give an added measure of authority and Oriental mystique to Atkinson's writings on yoga. There were also the aforementioned Western magicians who dressed in a variety of Oriental costumes during their performances.[82] In addition, there were those who took on Oriental identities because being fetishized was rather preferable to being lynched. Such was the story of one Reverend Jesse Wayman Routté, who donned velvet robes, a spangled purple turban, and his best Swedish accent to keep Jim Crow laws at bay on his trip through the American South in 1947, introducing himself as an "Apostle of Good Will and Love."[83] There were others who straddled the line between marketing tactics and defense mechanisms in their Yogi impersonations. For instance, Arthur Dowling, an African American vaudeville performer during the first two decades of the twentieth century, went by the stage name of Jovedah de Rajah and billed himself as "The East Indian Psychic."[84]

Yogi Panic

Of course, many Americans had been far more comfortable with Yogis when they remained on the printed page or at least on the vaudeville stage. Besides eliciting a general xenophobic discomfort that was associated with immigrants of any kind, Yogis presented a very particular problem. The issue was well articulated by a 1912 article in the *Washington Post*, aptly titled, "American Women Victims of Hindu Mysticism" (fig. 1.2), which, after a long exposition of the dangers of Indian religion and the terrible fates of women who had succumbed to its charms, concluded thus:

> The Hindu as a factor in the labor problem has so far not troubled the eastern United States, although he has been the cause of some trouble and rioting in the West. In New York city there are probably less than 50 Hindus, and most of these are at Columbia University and other institutions of learning.
>
> The Hindu problem of the east lies in the presence of the swamis, or teachers, educated and able men, who with their swarthy faces and dreamy-looking eyes stand in themselves symbolic of the mystery of the Orient. It is their teachings, their appeals for their disciples to try to attain impossible goals by unaccustomed paths that they are largely responsible for the deluded women who give away fortunes to "the cause," who give up home and children, and who, breaking down under the strain become hopeless lunatics.

This analysis came on the heels of a very public trial over the will of Sara Chapman Bull (1850–1911), a wealthy socialite whose Cambridge residence had a rotating door for Indian teachers and the Harvard intellectuals who wished to rub

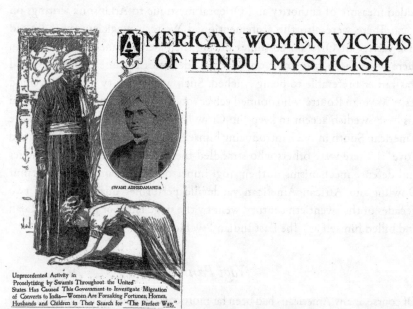

AMERICAN WOMEN VICTIMS OF HINDU MYSTICISM

SWAMI ABHEDANANDA

Unprecedented Activity in Proselytizing by Swamis Throughout the United States Has Caused This Government to Investigate Migration of Converts to India—Women Are Forsaking Fortunes, Homes, Husbands and Children in Their Search for "The Perfect Way."

FIGURE 1.2 "American Women Victims of Hindu Mysticism," *Washington Post*, February 12, 1912

shoulders with them. Bull, upon her death in 1911, left nearly all of her considerable estate to the Vedanta Society, a decision that her daughter was—for obvious reasons—less than elated about and chose to contest on the grounds that decades of interactions with Yogi teachers had driven her mother insane. Testimony to establish Bull's insanity ranged from her bizarre eating habits (a bit of milk and six almonds a day), to incense burning and alleged drug use, to participation in "love rites" and "delights of the love stage of yoga," the details of which were apparently so salacious as to be sealed by the court.[85]

The details that were revealed, however, demonstrate interesting insights into the ideas that were coming to be associated with yoga—or "yogi," which was regularly used to refer to both the practice and its practitioners. In addition to the scandalous activities described above, sources describe the practice of "Raja Yogi" as involving the awakening and ascension of the "Kundalina" (*kuṇḍalinī*) into the brain via the "sussuma" (*suṣumnā*) canal. Nicola Roberta, a student of Bull and subsequent witness in the case seeking to establish her insanity, testified that as part of the practice "we sat in a line or in a circle and breathed deeply. We tried to breathe entirely through the left nostril and concentrated on it until we felt the breath going way down to kindalina [base of spine]." Roberts also specified that this was accompanied by "exercises in the imagination" in which the practitioners would imagine "a locust on the top of our heads growing brighter and brighter or to imagine that there was a locust in our hearts growing brighter and brighter."[86] Despite the abundant and variable misspellings, the testimonies accurately describe a basic form of *prāṇāyāma* breathing exercise and meditative visualization, which is consistent with other reports of the contents of Vivekananda's teachings during his American tour. Of course, one certainly hopes that the "locust in our hearts" was a misunderstanding on the part of the *Chicago Tribune* reporter who recorded Roberta's description of the visualization rather than Roberta himself. A lotus is a traditional—and much more pleasant—image often invoked during meditative practice.

Regardless of their objective accuracy, the strangeness of the described practices no doubt contributed to the fervent panic over the dangers posed by Yogis. Bull's case was one of a number of such incidents that received considerable publicity during the first three decades of the twentieth century. Just before Bull, in 1910, there was Sarah Jane Farmer (1844–1916), who established a spiritual center in Maine following the 1893 World Parliament of Religions and hosted a large number of foreign as well as domestic metaphysical teachers and intellectuals. However, after she decided to join the Baha'i faith and leave much of her estate to a corresponding community, she was declared mentally incompetent and confined to an insane asylum by her heirs.[87]

Many similar stories litter the popular press of the time: In 1909, Yogi William F. Garnett, "seer and fortune teller," was charged with defrauding multiple women.[88] In 1910, "Hindu hypnotist" Sakharam G. Pandit was arrested for offering a woman a "massage treatment" as part of "Yogi religion."[89] In 1926, Annis Schuler, "a pretty Los Angeles matron" filed for divorce from her husband citing his keenness for "Yogi philosophy" as the reason. According to Mrs. Schuler, "as long as his pursuit of knowledge along Yogi philosophical lines was confined to various and sundry attempts to exercise hypnotism on her . . . it was not so bad, but— The incident of the housetop gymnastics in scanty attire with numerous neighbors as spectators not only caused her much mental anguish and suffering, . . . it brought her to the realization that philosophy of Yogi tendencies as practiced by her husband are incompatible with happy married life."[90] In 1935, Yogi Dassaunda Singh Roy was arrested and tried for distributing various herbal medicines, including alleged abortifacients, to several women.[91] The American public thus had plenty of material on the grounds of which Yogi teachers could be established as a looming threat. Although he initially seemed innocuous compared to his more ostentatious counterparts, the mystic was quickly becoming the most worrisome Yogi persona of all.

Indeed, as these examples demonstrate, anyone who called himself a Yogi posed a potential danger, regardless of whether he was Indian or not. Bernard, though decidedly American in origin, found himself at the center of the worst media circus to swallow up any other Yogi before him. Of course, Bernard was not altogether innocent. He had indeed been involved in sexual relationships with a number of his female disciples and when one of them testified that he had approached her saying 'I am not a real man. . . . I am a god, but I have condescended to put on the habit of a man, that I perform the duties of a yogi, and reveal true religion to the elect of America,"[92] there may have been more than a little truth to her story. The *Washington Post* article in which this claim appeared also intimated that Bernard had "induced her [Gertrude Leo] to come East with him by promise to give her free treatment." Thus, while Bernard may have in fact been a European American, this fact was either lost on the mass public or he possessed enough of an association with the Orient so that his actual ethnic identity did not much matter.

Furthermore, while Gertrude Leo may have been exploited to a certain degree, she did initially join Bernard's Order of her own accord. Similarly, while there is no way of determining exactly what had transpired between the two Sara(h)s— Bull and Farmer—and their teachers, leading them to disinherit their families in favor of their spiritual communities, it is likely that the two women had not in fact been driven to insanity as their heirs claimed. There is another story to be told here—one that deals with the dynamics of women's participation in metaphysical religious movements as part of the larger narrative of women's social and sexual liberation during the late nineteenth and early twentieth centuries. While a few studies have examined this phenomenon in the context of movements such as Spiritualism, Christian Science, and New Thought,[93] no extensive work has been done with regard to Asian-inspired movements and yoga.

The parties who were clutching their pearls over the exploitation of American women were far more concerned with the presumed active agents in this interaction: the Yogis. Anxiety over women's independence and trumped up panic over "white slavery"[94] led to a number of Yogis being charged with everything from sexual impropriety to hypnotism. Elizabeth A. Reed, whose voice proved particularly effective due to her position as a respected Orientalist scholar, claimed that "the Guru is a modern money-making invention"[95] who had long been preying on the credulity of India's women but has now brought the same strategies to America. She claimed that "the Swami, Gossian, or Guru is now quite at home in both Europe and America and many a desolated home lies in the trail of his silken robes,"[96] and further elaborated:

> In one of our great cities, the headquarters of a Hindu cult are, or were until very recently, in charge of an American woman who had taken the terrible vows, and the veil of an Indian nun.... A well-known New England woman, having fallen under the hypnotic say of a Swami, made over her entire fortune at his dictation. After the papers were safely made out, the "further mysteries" were revealed to her. Can we wonder that she then went hopelessly insane and was for years—in the asylum? ... One well-known Swami was in the habit of receiving the adoration of his followers, when he came out of his daily meditation. Then these American woman were ready to caress his robe, and kiss his sandaled feet.[97]

The image of American women bowing at and kissing the feet of their Indian masters proved so shocking for many Americans that it spread like wildfire as a symbol of the Yogi's power. Reed warns, "let the white woman beware of the hypnotic influence of the East—let her remember that when her Guru, or god-man, has once whispered his mystic syllables into her ear and she has sworn allegiance to him, she is forever helpless in his hands."[98] It is unclear how many American women took her words to heart, but it is clear that a number of American men did. For every account of a Yogi giving a celebrated lecture in a major American city, there is usually a corresponding account of him being chased out or being threatened by an army of angry husbands.

A number of other anti-Hindu publications emerged around this time, adding fuel to the xenophobic panic. Among these were Mabel Potter Dagget's "The Heathen Invasion" (1911), Mrs. Gross Alexander's "American Women Going after Heathen Gods" (1912),[99] Katherine Mayo's *Mother India* (1927), and Mersene

Sloan's *The Indian Menace* (1929). Of these, Mayo's work was distinctive in that it deals primarily with the state of things in India itself rather than with anything occurring on American soil. However, her representation of India as a land of filth, disease, and above all sexual perversion no doubt infected domestic visions of anyone and anything perceived as hailing from within its borders. Mayo was, like Reed, a historian whose academic credentials gave her voice amplified sway, and her book was a top-ten bestseller in 1927 and 1928.

With their unsavory reputation firmly in place, Yogis quickly became stock characters in Hollywood murder mysteries and dramas, with an occasional detour into comedy, through the first half of the twentieth century. The Yogi (or Swami) was often unnamed, almost always a fraud, and habitually engaged in murder, coerced suicide, illicit rituals, and deceiving of gullible women. The consistently suggestive titles include: *The Love Girl* (1916, see fig. 1.3), *Upside Down* (1919), *Thirteen Women* (1932), *Sinister Hands* (1932), *Sucker Money* (1933), *The Mind Reader* (1933), *Moonlight Murder* (1936), *Religious Racketeers* (1938), and *Bunco Squad* (1950).

Yet despite the very real legal and social consequences such characterizations had for those who wished to identify as Yogis, the mystique continued unabated. For every slew of angry husbands looking to chase the offending Swami out of town, there was the implied equally large slew of spiritually seeking wives who were only too eager to receive what the mystic might have to offer. This is not to say that the Yogi's followers (or victims, as popular opinion would have it) were always women, though photographs of lectures and other gatherings do reveal a sizeable female majority. However, as in many instances, cultural anxieties were far more effectively played out on female bodies and psyches.

As the cases of Bull and Farmer demonstrate, women who earnestly and agentively pursued their interest in yogic ideas and practice were subject to aggressive forms of social sanction. While Bull was deceased by the time that legal measures were brought to undermine her will and Farmer, though institutionalized, was eventually liberated by members of her community, not all women were so lucky. The most drastic example is perhaps that of Ida B. Craddock, a prominent occultist, women's rights activist, and sex reform advocate. Craddock, who opened her own Church of Yoga in 1899, was imprisoned under the era's strict anti-obscenity laws and committed suicide before facing her federal trial.[100] Craddock is significant in other ways, none the least of which is her incorporation of dance into her understanding of yoga. She is one in an entire line of "dancing girls"—Bernard's wife De Vries is another prominent example—who would gradually take over and transform the face of postural yoga in the United States as immigration restrictions stymied the influx of Indian Yogis. This would bring about a profound transformation in the form and public visibility of physical practice. After all,

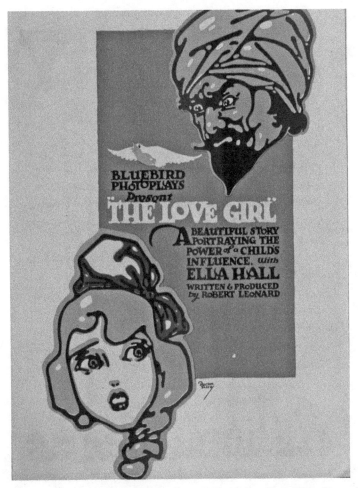

FIGURE 1.3 Film advertisement for *The Love Girl* (1916) in *The Moving Picture World*, July 1916

postures that read as bizarre contortions when enacted by South Asian male bodies easily transitioned into aesthetically appropriate gymnastics when translated onto white female bodies.

However, it would be a few decades before Americans would be ready to view white women as fully competent and self-possessed students and teachers of yoga. Just as naturally passive and suggestible women had served as perfect vessels for the ghosts of Spiritualism, so they became ideal subjects for the Yogi's hypnotic powers. Ultimately these two phenomena were more than a little related, and thus it is to the metaphysical foundations of the Yogi's perceived powers that we will now turn.

2

Yogis Without Borders

By what power is this Akasha manufactured into this universe? By the power of Prana. Just as Akasha is the infinite, omnipresent material of this universe, so is this Prana the infinite, omnipresent manifesting power of this universe. At the beginning and at the end of a cycle everything becomes Akasha, and all the forces that are in the universe resolve back into the Prana; in the next cycle, out of this Prana is evolved everything that we call energy, everything that we call force. . . . When the Yogi becomes perfect, there will be nothing in nature not under his control. If he orders the gods or the souls of the departed to come, they will come at his bidding. All the forces of nature will obey him as slaves. When the ignorant see these powers of the Yogi, they call them the miracles.

—VIVEKANANDA, *Raja Yoga*

What has the future in store for this strange being, born of a breath, of perishable tissue, yet Immortal, with his powers fearful and Divine? What magic will be wrought by him in the end? What is to be his greatest deed, his crowning achievement? Long ago he recognized that all perceptible matter comes from a primary substance, or a tenuity beyond conception, filling all space, the Akasha or luminiferous ether, which is acted upon by the life-giving Prana or Creative Force, calling into existence, in never ending cycles, all things and phenomena. . . . Can man control this grandest, most awe-inspiring of all processes in nature? Can he harness her inexhaustible energies to perform all their functions at his bidding, more still—cause them to operate simply by the force of his will? If he could do this, he would have powers almost unlimited and supernatural. At his command, with but a slight effort on his part, old worlds would disappear and new ones of his planning would spring into being.

—NIKOLA TESLA, "Man's Greatest Achievement"

IN THE PREVIOUS chapter, we encountered some early modern Yogis and observed as their stories gradually filtered into the Western imagination. This chapter concerns itself largely with the ideological mechanisms of this latter process. Specifically, it explores the metaphysical and philosophical underpinnings of the Yogi's persona and power. In order for the Yogi to enter the Western imagination, his powers had to be comprehensible to the Western mindset. Here the focus is less on popular conceptions of the Yogi as a wielder of superpowers but rather on the elite metaphysical understandings, mainly by insiders of metaphysical thought, for the basis of these powers. In the popular arena, attributions of psychic or hypnotic ability—however "mystical"—are ultimately inherited from some basic understanding of this metaphysical schema.

Vivekananda's message caught on in no small part because the particular philosophy he was espousing picked up on the same flavor of metaphysical spirituality that was already well developed in the communities that received him. By the 1890s Spiritualism, with its sonic manifestations and ectoplasmic apparitions, had swept over the parlors of American homes,[1] and mind cure ideology was evident not only in the burgeoning traditions of New Thought and Christian Science but also in the growing popularity of therapeutic psychology.[2] Vivekananda generally rebuked calls to "put up or shut up"[3] with respect to displays of superhuman power. However, that his authenticity and value should be judged by the ability to produce "miracles" testifies to the fact that in the American popular imagination—as in the Indian—the Yogi was first and foremost the man with superpowers.

The previous chapter concerned itself for the most part with how American audiences saw the Yogi. This chapter, on the other hand, will be concerned with how they understood him. In other words, it examines the history of ideas by means of which the Yogi's superpowers could be rendered not only comprehensible but justifiable in the face of modern scientific rationalism—a history that resulted in the meeting of minds between an Indian Swami (Vivekananda) and a Serbian-American engineer (Nikola Tesla) and that yielded the strikingly similar epigraphs that preface this section. The Yogi's ability to be comprehensible as anything other than a caricature required that the powers that lay at the root of his identity be represented in manner that was intelligible to his audience. For instance, as we have seen, when faced with the seemingly magical abilities of exotic Yogis and fakirs, Western observers often appealed to the power of hypnotism, which rendered their performances more realistically palatable. After all, in a culture enthusiastically beginning to discover the powers of the human mind, believing that an audience was hypnotized into seeing a boy climbing a levitating rope only to disappear into nothing required less of a mental stretch than believing that the rope really levitated and the boy really disappeared. However, even hypnotism ultimately begged for an explanation, and stories of more physically grounded phenomena continued to filter into the public imagination. Whether the Yogi—or the more domestic Spiritualist medium—actually controlled physical reality or simply its perception in the minds of others, the mechanisms of his method still required elucidation.

Ultimately the vision of the Yogi as a superpowerful mystic proved appealing because it was an alluringly exotic but ultimately familiar instantiation of an already pervasive Western trope of the perfected human being. Emerging out of the perfectionistic concerns of Western esotericism and alchemy, this notion of the superman, glorified in Friedrich Nietzsche's *Thus Spoke Zarathustra* (1891), manifested its darker side in the eugenics fervor and Social Darwinism movement of the late nineteenth century. As has been argued by Mark Singleton, the growing enterprise of modern yoga was by no means uninvolved in these developments.[4] In American metaphysical spirituality, however, the notion of human perfection took on a sunnier disposition and a more optimistic tone aimed at healing and the transcendence of human limitations. The Yogi found himself quite at home amidst those tributaries of the modern New Age movement that ultimately focus on what Paul Heelas has identified as "Self-spirituality," or the divinization of the human self.[5] In the figure of the Yogi rested a concrete example—supported by millennia of "Oriental" wisdom—of the cosmic destiny of human potential. Only a year after the publication of Vivekananda's *Raja Yoga* (1896), Ralph Waldo Trine's wildly popular *In Tune with the Infinite* (1897) would proclaim that "in the degree that we open ourselves to this divine inflow are we changed from mere men into God-men."[6]

In Trine's words, we see the second half of the superhuman equation. Human evolution, whether it be understood materially or spiritually, could not be rendered intelligible without a complementary vision of the cosmos that could accommodate the superhuman telos. If humans can become superpowerful, it is only by means of approaching the ultimate reservoir of that power, the cosmos itself, and if evolution is a fundamentally natural process, then the cosmos has to hold a natural answer to the forces that seem profoundly supernatural. Catherine Albanese, who has given us the most thorough historical account and theoretical understanding of the purview of metaphysical traditions to date,[7] has stated that

> for metaphysical believers everything is linked to everything else—cut of the same cloth, as it were—and in metaphysics life becomes holographic. One piece of the universe can operate or act on any other piece of the universe, and, with the guiding power of Mind for steerage, seemingly miraculous change can become common-place and ordinary.[8]

But what is this "cloth"? Depending on the particular school of metaphysics, it might ultimately come down to God, or Spirit, or Mind. For Albanese, the least common denominator of metaphysical discourse is best articulated through the language of "energy" and "flow." She briefly notes that this energetic model generally conforms to scientific theories of ether in the nineteenth century before adopting the paradigms of quantum physics in the twentieth.

Although the language of waves, currents, magnetism, and electricity is fairly ubiquitous across metaphysical literature, regardless of the particular tradition to which it belongs, some authors take this terminology more literally than others. Indeed, these scientific metaphors are so pervasive precisely because the development of post-Enlightenment metaphysical traditions has historically hewed quite closely to the development of post-Enlightenment science. The energetic models of metaphysical traditions like Mesmerism, Spiritualism, Theosophy, and to a lesser extent Christian Science and New Thought, do not simply resemble scientific theories of ether; they frequently rely on and directly co-opt these theories. There exists a blurry line between physics and metaphysics, demonstrated by the reliance on popular scientific theory even by more esoteric metaphysical schools such as Theosophy, and this line becomes progressively blurrier the further back one follows it in time.

This chapter seeks to elucidate two points. On the one hand, it argues that scientific theory has consistently served as a crucial element of metaphysical thought and, indeed, that the two have often functioned in tandem. To this end, it offers an alternative and complementary reading of the evolution of metaphysical spirituality in the United States by shifting the focus from the spiritual force of mind to its metaphysical medium—the ether. In doing so, it sheds new light on the relationship between metaphysical religion and modernity, especially in the form of scientific rationalism, that has been the focus of so many previous studies.

On the other hand, this chapter traces the history of a single set of analogous terms—English *ether* and Sanskrit *ākāśa*—as a way of illustrating just how inextricably intertwined Indian and Western categories of thought can become when they enter the dialogue of metaphysical speculation. From one perspective, one might say that the pull of modern rationalism was so strong, both among the intelligentsia of colonial India and in the West, that Indian categories adapted by reemerging as Western scientific concepts in disguise. However, the real dynamic is far more complicated, as the Western appropriation and Indian reappropriation of such categories reflect an ongoing contestation of spheres of value and authority. The dialogic nature of the relationship is crucial to note. The association of *ākāśa* with ether opened a linguistic door by way of which Vivekananda's modernized Yogi was able to enter Western metaphysical thought, but the entrance of the Yogi in turn reinforced the individualistic yet universal flavor of the metaphysical discourse of human potential. A scientifically rationalized Yogi—at once Self and Other, familiar yet strange, embodied in the human (Indian) man and yet somehow beyond even him—transformed the occult ascended master into a self-realized Everyman.

The few existing histories of ether tend to tread on the side of either the purely scientific or the strictly occult and spiritual. This is most likely due in large part to an understandable disciplinary divide, but the truth of the matter is that many of the same individuals who were involved in developing theories of ether(s) as "scientific" concepts were also deeply invested in theorizing the possible functions of these substances as spiritual media. Ether and *ākāśa* first came together in the translations of early Indologists. As we will see, there are undeniable analogies between the two terms that justify this move. However, translation is always situated in and therefore inseparable from the historical and ideological context of the translator and thus can have a way of investing terms with baggage that is not historically their own. In the case of *ākāśa*, this baggage came not only in the form of Western esotericism but also contemporary scientific associations. Consequently, even as the Theosophists adopted and popularized *ākāśa* as an exotic Oriental form of their occult subtle materiality, they cleared the space for this Indian metaphysical concept to become an elaboration of the theorized scientific entity that the occult mirrors. Vivekananda relied extensively on these linkages in his work, and he was by no means the last Indian teacher to do so. The final portion of this chapter illustrates the ways in which an occultized ether entered the age of quantum theory in the works of another Indian Swami, Paramahansa Yogananda, who effectively took up Vivekananda's mantle as the popular embodiment of the Yogi in America.

Ākāśa, or Akasha as it is usually rendered in English, is certainly not found in the colloquial Sanskrit vocabulary, consisting of "naturalized" terms like karma, nirvana, guru, and so on, which are generally recognized by most culturally savvy Westerners. However, the sudden appearance of this term in metaphysical texts during the period that marks the introduction of Indian thought into Western metaphysical spirituality is a smoking gun that testifies to the importance of the concept that it represents. In other words, we cannot understand the full metaphysical significance of the more pervasively used "ether" until we examine the moment at which it became "*ākāśa*."

The latter term now survives largely in the Theosophical tradition that first introduced it into the West as well as in the Theosophical Society's offshoots, such as Rudolf Steiner's Anthroposophy and the work of Alice A. Bailey. In these contexts, *ākāśa* manifests as the "Akashic Record," an increasingly immaterial concept that refers to the cosmic repository of all human knowledge and experience. In the realm of popular culture, *ākāśa* flits furtively into and out of view whenever a sufficiently mystically charged term is in order. It appears, for instance, as the name of the ancient Egyptian queen from whom all of Anne

Rice's literary vampires are descended. It should be noted that in Rice's work vampires are stunningly attractive superhumans—one might say perfected beings—who eventually develop abilities such as telepathy, telekinesis, and flight. So there is that.

Ākāśa *in India*

Because of the richness of Indian theories dealing with subtle materiality and embodiment—a richness whose scope cannot be adequately represented within the confines of this chapter—I will leave aside an elaboration of these larger frameworks and focus instead on the specific signifier of *ākāśa*, which comes to largely represent these various modalities as they make their way into the West. In its generic sense, *ākāśa* can be translated as "space," "atmosphere," or "sky." Of course, it can acquire a range of more specialized meanings depending on context. Of these, perhaps the most useful for the purposes of this chapter is its role as cosmological element. In the context of Indian philosophical discourse, *ākāśa* appears in the treatises of Sāṃkhya and Nyāya-Vaiśeṣika as well as in Jain and Buddhist metaphysics. In Sāṃkhya and Nyāya-Vaiśeṣika, *ākāśa* is commonly established as the substratum for sound, though the particularities of its nature vary. Because Vedāntin metaphysics—on which Vivekananda and other modern exponents of Indian thought overwhelmingly draw—primarily co-opts the framework of the classical Sāṃkhyan system, I will not go into the details of Nyāya-Vaiśeṣika's conception of *ākāśa*, other than to note that it differs chiefly in that it presents *ākāśa*, unlike the other four elements (*vāyu* or air, *tejas* or fire, *ap* or water, and *pṛthivī* or earth), as non-atomic and eternal (*nitya*).[9] In the Sāṃkhyan schema, all five gross elements (*mahābhūtas*) are considered to be evolutes of the five subtle elements (*tanmātras*), which are in turn evolutes of the hierarchical sequence of principles (*tattvas*) stemming from the unmanifest substratum of material nature (*mūlaprakṛti*). Here *ākāśa* is notable for two reasons: it is the subtlest of the five *mahābhūtas*, and consequently it is commonly seen as giving rise to the other four, thereby possessing a creative quality.[10]

Turning particularly to yogic traditions, we find that *ākāśa* is often present but never a central point of concern. In the context of Pātañjala yoga, which roughly follows Sāṃkhyan metaphysics, *ākāśa* does not appear to play any special role, besides being instrumental in the attainment of the ever-coveted *siddhi* (superpower) of flight. *Yoga Sūtra* 3.42 states that sustained meditation (*saṃyama*) on the relationship between *ākāśa* and the body (*kāyākāśayoḥ sambandha*) results in the ability to travel through the same *ākāśa* (*ākāśagamanam*). There are quite a few significant resonances to be found between the general concept of ether or space and yogic attainment in the context of later tantric traditions, but these tend to more frequently employ synonymous terminology such as *vyoman*, *gagana*, and *kha*.[11]

Thus, although *ākāśa* is certainly pervasive as both a term and general concept in Indian understandings of subtle embodiment and metaphysics, it constitutes only a minor component of these schemas. It is generally understood as only a single element of a larger framework and is only rarely envisioned as being anywhere near the originating basis of material reality at large. When it is used in a more generic sense, it can become descriptive of or even synonymous with aspects of absolute reality, but in these cases it loses its material quality, coming instead to represent the uniquely non-material character of the absolute.

Although Indian notions of subtle materiality certainly come to be assimilated into Western conceptions of the same, when we encounter the specific term *ākāśa*, it tends to assume something other than its original role. In responding to the Western framework of mind-body dualism, which associates mind with spirit and body with matter, both the Theosophists' and Vivekananda's schemas yield conflicting visions of what constitutes materiality. Following Sāṃkhyan and Vedāntin conceptions of *ākāśa* as the source of the other gross elements, both tend to equate the term with the source of materiality writ-large. The position of the mind and its constituent *tattva*s thus becomes ambiguous, since such principles are considered aspects of materiality in the original Indian framework but not in the Western context into which they are introduced. Thus, *ākāśa*, conforming to its analogous ethereal counterpart, at times comes to signify the bridge between materiality and the mind, which is not quite spirit but is no longer matter as such.

Western Theories of Ether

The Western side of this early history begins, as things usually do in mainstream narratives of Western civilization, with the ancient Greeks. Concepts of *aer* (atmospheric misty air) and *aither* (a shining, blazing, fiery upper air) were employed in the metaphysics of sixth-century BCE Ionian philosophers in ways that indicate an already well-established common cosmological understanding. These two entities could be interpreted in variable ways along with a third, *pneuma* (the air of breath), to yield something like an ethereal cosmogony.[12] However, it is not until the work of Aristotle that we see a full theory of ether. For Aristotle, the fifth element of the celestial *aither*—the other four being air, fire, water, and earth—has an earthly analog in the circulation of the animating force of *pneuma*, or life breath. The Stoics go on to equate the two, further associating them with the embodiment of the active principle of *logos*, which penetrates and acts upon matter to effect creation. The mechanics of this embodiment and action are, however, never fully elaborated.[13]

No significant developments in the metaphysical status of ether occur until the concept reappears in the work of René Descartes (1596–1650), who proposed the existence of three elements, generally identified with fire, air, and earth, though not to be equated with their conventionally acknowledged physical manifestations. Movements of particles of the first element constitute heat. When these additionally exert pressure on and effect movement in the particles of the second element, the pressure transmitted by this interaction results in light. For Descartes, subtle matter, which serves as the medium for light and is identified with ether, comprises the second element permeated by the first. In turn, any changes observed in gross material bodies composed of the third element can be traced back to interactions with this subtle materiality.[14] G. N. Cantor and M. J. S. Hodge, in tracing the history of theories of ether, argue that although it is generally maintained that Descartes's ethereal hypotheses were "highly speculative" and that their "main influence was in convincing people of the coherence of mechanical explanation in general," many of the subsequent breakthroughs that inaugurate the emergence of modern scientific theories can be linked to acceptance, rejection, or modification of his proposals.[15] Even the work of Isaac Newton (1642–1727), who largely distanced himself from both mechanical philosophy in general and Descartes in particular, cannot be interpreted without reference to the latter.

Newton, that famous father of modern physics, was also largely responsible for the theory of the luminiferous, or "light-bearing," ether that would remain generally accepted in scientific circles well into the late nineteenth century. Keeping in mind that physics and metaphysics have not always shared the strictly delineated border they do today, it might be safely said that in the eighteenth and nineteenth centuries ether was primarily a scientific concept. In fact, Newton theorized several different ethers, which were not always altogether consistent with each other. Chief among these were theories of ether as a medium for the propagation of electromagnetic and gravitational forces. Newton was not always clear on the nature of this proposed ether, and in his second published paper on optics actually suggested that rather than constituting "one uniform matter" it was in fact a combination of "the main phlegmatic body of aether," which was inactive, with active and subtler "aetherial spirits."[16] He further suggested that this mixture could be condensed to produce diverse forms of matter. Newton even went so far as to suggest in an unpublished version of the manuscript of his third volume of *Opticks* that electricity could be equated with the subtle spirit that produced all natural phenomena.[17]

Newton's theory of the ether in relation to light, which he understood as made of corpuscular particles rather than a wave akin to heat radiation, was actually substantially divergent from later understandings. Nevertheless, by suggesting that the refraction of light particles occurred due to interference of an ethereal medium, he established the basis for his successors to hypothesize that it was exactly this medium through which the newly established transverse wave of light must travel. This remained the reigning theory among physicists—even as several sets of experiments conducted in the late nineteenth century proved it untenable by failing to discover any such substance—until the need for it was gradually eliminated by the advent and acceptance of quantum mechanics.[18] However, even as ether continued to pervade the atmosphere of theoretical physics, it also caught on in other circles. Indeed, Newton introduced a variety of functions for his ether(s) that prefigure the various universal magnetic fluids that would later be used to explain the phenomena of the pseudo-medical tradition of Mesmerism and its more popular offspring, Spiritualism.[19]

Magnetic Bodies and Mesmeric Trances

These connections are not at all coincidental, as Franz Anton Mesmer (1734–1815) was decidedly a student of Newton's work. Mesmer, borrowing heavily from Newton's more metaphysically inclined theories, set out to instrumentalize them in the sphere of medicine. Mesmer's dissertation, *Dissertatio Physico-medica de Planetarum Influxu* (1766), built on—or possibly plagiarized from—the ideas of Richard Mead, a prominent English physician, and adapted Newton's hypotheses to argue that bodies were universally subject to an all-pervading gravitation emanating from the stars. He referred to this principle as "animal gravitation," the predecessor to his famous concept of animal magnetism.

In his subsequent medical practice, Mesmer experimented with using iron magnets to treat illness, relying on the assumption that disease was caused by a body's having fallen out of harmony with a universal force, which was no longer based solely on gravitation in relation to heavenly bodies but also emanating from and pervading animal bodies. The initial stages of this therapy approached the aforementioned theory from a very literal perspective, as patients swallowed a solution containing traces of iron before having magnets placed on their bodies to redirect and thereby recalibrate the flow of their vital magnetic energies. Mesmer did not generally employ the language of ether in his work, but nevertheless spoke of a "fluid which is universally widespread and pervasive in a manner which allows for no void, subtly permits no comparison, and is of a nature which is susceptible to receive, propagate, and communicate all impressions of movement."[20] He analogized the operation of this force to the manipulation of both magnetism and electricity, but insisted that the latter were only naturally differentiated manifestations of a universal force that lay at the root of all phenomena. Moreover, if Mesmer himself did not make this metaphysical association explicit, it was almost certainly understood as such by his audience.

In keeping with this line of reasoning, Mesmer eventually concluded that the physical instrument of the magnet was secondary—and eventually superfluous—to the real instrument through which magnetic healing was effected: the person of the magnetist himself. External props were not altogether abandoned. Mesmer introduced the somewhat more imposing device of the *baquet*, which constituted a sort of large wooden tub filled with jars of "magnetized" water set upon metal filings. Patients would be connected to and thereby able to access the concentrated magnetic fluid stored in the device by virtue of metal rods extending out of the periphery of the container's lid. Not to be outdone by his device, Mesmer contributed to the theatrical atmosphere by donning a lilac taffeta robe and, thus raimented, would generate further "sanative" vibrations by playing on a glass harmonica or sashaying from one patient to the next brandishing a wand.[21]

Despite his best efforts, Mesmer's technique failed to win the approval of the medical community. In 1784 a special Royal Commission charged with investigating his work (and decorated with such notable members as Benjamin Franklin) failed to find any merit in his endeavors. After this Mesmer's personal popularity declined, and he spent the remainder of his days in relative obscurity. However, the larger tradition of Mesmerism was far from dead. After Mesmer's retreat from the public arena, the term "Mesmerism" took on a somewhat different connotation, chiefly propagated by his most notable disciple, the Marquis de Puységur, Amand Marie Jacques de Chastenet (1751–1825). In Puységur's work, Mesmerism was dissociated from all use of external props and became tied primarily to a somnambulistic altered state, often accompanied by clairvoyance. In this form, Mesmerism would persist in three essential forms: the medical, the psychological, and the parapsychological.[22]

It is the latter parapsychological stream than most concerns our subject matter here, but a note should be made about an interesting and often ignored association between it and its more traditionally psychological cousin. Puységur's work was monumentally influential in the development of hypnotism, which accounts for much of Mesmerism's presence in the sphere of psychology. The term "hypnotism," originally "neuro-hypnotism," was coined by Scottish physician James Braid (1795–1860) in 1842 as an alternative to the terminology of animal magnetism. Unlike Puységur, Braid completely divorced the mechanics of Mesmerism from any association with a universal magnetic fluid and described it as an exclusively psychological phenomenon, hence the change in nomenclature.

However, although in its properly historical context hypnotism is simply a more metaphysically conservative derivative of Mesmerism and the two terms sometimes continue to be used synonymously, their differentiation may take on an entirely different set of valences in metaphysical and occult circles. For instance, Helena Blavatsky, in responding to a query on how one should differentiate between Mesmerism (or magnetism) and hypnotism, purports to quote the work of French psychologist Amédée H. Simonin in his *Solution du problème de la suggestion hypnotique* (1889) to explain that

> while "in Magnetism (mesmerism) there occurs in the subject a great development of moral faculties"; that his thoughts and feelings "become loftier, and the senses acquire an abnormal acuteness"; in hypnotism, on the contrary, "the subject becomes a simple mirror."
>
>   . . .
>
> "In hypnotism instinct, i.e., the animal, reaches its greatest development; so much so, indeed, that the aphorism 'extremes meet' can never receive a better application than to magnetism and hypnotism." How true these words, also, as to the difference between the mesmerized and the hypnotized subjects. "In one, his ideal nature, his moral self—the reflection of his divine nature—are carried to their extreme limits, and the subject becomes almost a celestial being (un ange). In the other, it is his instincts which develop in a most surprising fashion. The hypnotic lowers himself to the level of the animal. From a physiological standpoint, magnetism ('Mesmerism') is comforting and curative, and hypnotism, which is but the result of an unbalanced state, is—most dangerous."[23]

It should be noted that no passages that could yield the above translations actually appear in Simonin's original French. Nevertheless, Blavatsky's (invented) references reflect an appraisal of the respective connotations of Mesmerism as opposed to hypnotism and the relative merit of their associated practices that must have been current in Theosophical as well as broader metaphysical circles.

It is notable that some forty years later Yogananda, when accused of hypnotism by an outraged Miami police chief, argued that he practiced magnetism, which was to be seen as an entirely different matter. Swami Kriyananda (1926–2013), a Westerner who was one of Yogananda's most fervent direct disciples, describes "magnetism" as a force that is

> generated by the amount and quality of the energy one projects. And this energy depends on the strength of a person's will power. "The greater the will," was Yogananda's frequently iterated maxim, "the greater the flow of

energy." . . . Success in every aspect of life depends on the strength of a person's magnetism to attract it.[24]

Thus, magnetism, in Yogananda's interpretation, loses all association with its mesmeric origins and becomes instead a metaphysical principle of personal will akin to a strengthened form of the Law of Attraction as it was espoused in contemporary New Thought circles.[25]

Although Yogananda's version of magnetism seems at first glance to be totally divorced from its roots in Mesmer's principle of animal magnetism, the two phenomena share a crucial commonality. Mesmer's own practice, despite its somewhat ignoble end, is significant precisely in its attempted synthesis of the occult with the scientific. Notwithstanding his fervent assertions that there was nothing "supernatural" or "magical" about his method, Mesmer's eccentric presentation, lilac robe and all, was clearly meant to lend a degree of mystique to the proceedings. While this aura of esotericism only aided in discrediting Mesmer's technique as parlor charlatanism in the eyes of the scientific community, it reflected a key element of how Mesmer viewed himself in relation to the technique. He was the modern magus turned scientist—an adept who had mastered control over a mystical but thoroughly natural universal principle that held the key to the most fundamental aspects of material reality.

The most notable manifestation of "parapsychological" Mesmerism can be found in American Spiritualism, which eventually closed the loop by returning to the European parlors that first nurtured its previous incarnation. The American mesmeric boom began in 1836 when Charles Poyen, a French disciple of the Marquis de Puységur, began a lecture tour across New England. By 1843 there were two hundred mesmerists practicing in the Boston area alone.[26] While much of American Mesmerism took the form of traveling mesmerists who would earn their living by diagnosing illnesses through clairvoyant somnambulism, a more cosmically expansive strand soon began to gain momentum. This was chiefly owed to the influence of Swedenborgian cosmologies, which provided an effective map to a multi-leveled universe populated with spirits possessed of various degrees of development. Emmanuel Swedenborg (1688–1772), a celebrated Swedish mystic and seer, left behind a voluminous body of publications cataloguing his trance-state journeys into celestial and infernal realms as well as the diverse planets of the known cosmos. While Swedenborg himself advised great caution in communing with spirits and ultimately insisted that it was the exclusive role of the spiritual adept—meaning himself—to engage in such potentially perilous otherworldly contact, his experiential narratives and theological tracts ultimately became blueprints for an unprecedented level of popular trance practice.

This mystical brand of Mesmerism had already begun to develop among the German Romantics of the early nineteenth century. German physician Johann Heinrich Jung-Stilling (1740–1817) fused notions of animal magnetism, Swedenborgian cosmology, and contemporary scientific theory to postulate a psychic body whose substance was composed of the luminiferous ether.[27] In America, the efforts of phrenomagnetists—individuals who yoked mesmeric somnambulism with the cranial analysis and manipulation of phrenology—such as John Bovee Dods (1795–1872), Joseph Rhodes Buchanan (1814–1899), and La Roy Sunderland (1802–1885), created a theoretical framework of mesmeric practice that affectively accommodated spiritual intervention.[28] By the time that the now-famous Fox sisters heard the mysterious rappings at their home in western New York in 1848, thus inaugurating the rise of the Spiritualist movement proper,[29] the metaphysical framework to explain these phenomena was conveniently at the ready.

One primary distinction between the mechanics of Mesmerism and Spiritualism lies in the role of the medium, who replaced the mesmerized patient. While mediums were by definition considered to be passive vessels through which spirits could speak—and indeed women were considered to be far more disposed to mediumistic talent specifically due to their docility—they did not strictly require an operator. That is, their trance states could and often were entirely self-induced. Indeed, scientists who exhibited an interest in mediumistic phenomena were far more likely to attribute their mechanics to the power of living medium than to the spirits of the deceased.[30] Whether it was the supranormal biology of ectoplasm, which yielded theories of "a vibratory organism that paralleled the ethereal undulations of the universe"[31] or the Spiritualistic uses of electrical discharge[32] such explanations tended to closely follow theories of ether. This was not necessarily a new development in the mesmeric community, as Braid had made a similar point in differentiating his psychological concept of hypnosis from the older and more physiological theories of animal magnetism. However, the Spiritualist medium possessed a very particular kind of agency that the mesmeric patient did not.[33]

The Theosophists, whose founders quite significantly emerged out of Spiritualist circles, would later take issue with the medium's subjection to the spirits whom she contacted. However, the independent clairvoyance of the medium was already a significant departure from the strict division of labor between the mesmeric adept and his dependently clairvoyant patient. One should nevertheless not overstate the medium's control over her own trance state. While there appears to have been a small minority of mediums who exhibited no marked changes in state of consciousness or personality and could in fact recall everything that had transpired while they were in trance, for the vast majority mediumship entailed a total break from their conventional subjectivity. At best, the medium was unique in her talent to submit herself to being directly mesmerized by subtle spirits rather than relying on a human operator.

Another related and perhaps even more significant innovation of Spiritualism was its accessibility to the common and even casual practitioner. Mediumship was generally considered to be a very specific kind of talent, of which a particular—often gender-specific—temperament was an accepted indicator. However, the practice of Spiritualism was not limited to professional mediums. Parlor séances often relied on the assumption that every human being possessed the energetic capacity for some mediumistic activity. Popular practices such as table tipping and various simplified forms of automatic writing (which yielded the now-trademarked Ouija board)[34] did not necessarily rely on the talent of a single medium but rather on the (meta)physical principle of a universal substratum of magnetic energy that the participants could tap into in order to either contact the spirit world or even manipulate the energies to directly effect the desired phenomenon. Thus, the popularity of Spiritualism largely relied on the assumption that every human being possessed the natural ability to interact with cosmic forces. While this ability manifested with greater strength in certain personalities, it was grounded in the inherent energetic potential of every human mind-body complex.

Theosophical Mahatmas Take Control

It is against this background that Theosophy emerged as both an organization and a body of thought. Inaugurated in a small New York City apartment on September 18, 1875, the Theosophical Society was co-founded by Henry Steel Olcott (1832–1907), an eclectic member of the New York urban gentry, and Helena Petrovna Blavatsky (1831–1891), a Bohemian expatriate of the Russian aristocracy. Both had had extensive ties with the Spiritualist movement.

Olcott, who had been a founding member of the New York Conference of Spiritualists, nevertheless grew increasingly ambivalent about the merits of Spiritualist phenomena. In an intellectual climate where "will"-based movements such as New Thought and other assorted strains of mind-cure were quickly gaining ascendancy and more established traditions such as Christian Science were continually cautioning against "Malicious Animal Magnetism," the medium held a precarious position. In an 1874 investigation of Spiritualistic phenomena, Olcott observed the following:

> The relation of the mediums towards their controlling spirits is perfectly defined in this letter from one of the most noted mediums—they are

slaves. While "under control," their own will is set aside, and their actions, their speech, and their very consciousness, are directed by that of another. They are helpless to do, or say, or think, or see what they desire, as the subject of the mesmerist, whose body is a mere machine governed by a will external to and dominant over itself. The "materializing medium" must even, it appears, lend from the more ethereal portions of his frame, some of the matter that goes to form the evanescent materialized shapes of the departed.[35]

In contrast to this assessment, Olcott referred to Blavatsky, whom he had only recently met at a Spiritualist demonstration in Chittendom, Vermont, as "one of the most remarkable mediums in the world" but qualified that "her mediumship is totally different from that of any other person I have ever met; for, instead of being controlled by spirits to do their will, it is she who seems to control them to do her bidding." This he attributes to Blavatsky's lengthy sojourn in "Oriental lands" where "what we recognize as Spiritualism, has for years been regarded as the mere rudimentary developments of a system which seems to have established such relations between mortals and the immortals as to enable certain of the former to have dominion over many of the latter."[36]

Blavatsky does appear to have traveled extensively between leaving her newly acquired husband, the vice-governor Nikifor Vladimirovich Blavatsky, in 1849 and turning up in New York in 1873. However, her exact itinerary during this lengthy period is largely uncorroborated and, while not strictly impossible, it is highly unlikely that a single white woman did in fact hike through the mountains of Tibet for several years in the mid-nineteenth century. Regardless of whether she had in fact ever set foot on South Asian soil prior to 1886, when she and Olcott relocated the Society's headquarters from New York to Adyar in Chennai, Blavatsky was singlehandedly responsible for opening the floodgates of Indian metaphysical categories that over the next century would thoroughly suffuse Western metaphysical spirituality. Reciprocally, however, these same categories would return to the source in the writings of Indian Theosophists—or even more numerous Theosophical sympathizers—laden with new Western valences. Such was the story of ākāśa, to which we shall return shortly.

Blavatsky's command of Oriental wisdom was famously credited to a brotherhood of Masters—or Mahatmas, as they would later come to be called—whose presence spanned all the nations and ages of human civilization. When Blavatsky was not communing with the Masters through automatic writing, to which she attributes much of her literary corpus, they would communicate through letters "precipitated" from the ceiling as they materialized out of the subtle etheric realms. It should be noted that despite her appeals to the mysteries of the Orient, Blavatsky did not romanticize its actual inhabitants. On the subject of Yogis, she had the following to say:

> A Yogi in India is a very elastic word. It now serves generally to designate a very dirty, dung-covered and naked individual, who never cuts nor combs his hair, covers himself from forehead to heels with wet ashes, performs Pranayam, without realizing its true meaning, and lives upon alms. It is only occasionally that the name is applied to one who is worthy of the appellation.[37]

The true Yogi, according to Blavatsky, was one who had achieved the original meaning of the term's etymology and, having renounced the transient pleasures of the world, had joined his soul with the great "Universal Soul." Under such circumstances, the Yogi could be considered identical to the Mahatma. However, not all Mahatmas were Yogis. Indeed, not all Mahatmas were Indian. Blavatsky's involvement with Indian thought grew through the course of her work, but her first Theosophical publication, *Isis Unveiled* (1877), relied much more heavily on Western esotericism and the work of such contemporary mystics as the French occultist Eliphas Levi (1810–1875), incorporating only fragments of Indian borrowings. Even as time went on, though Blavatsky missed no opportunity to invoke the spiritual authority of India, she and her associates were careful to maintain that their society was interested in propagating a universal truth rather than a sectarian religion. Indeed, Olcott maintains that this commitment to objectivity was responsible for the Theosophists' rocky three-year association and subsequent rupture with the neo-Hindu reform movement, the Ārya Samāj.

The mission statement of the Theosophical Society, as articulated by Olcott, was to offer an alternative to both "theological superstition" and "tame subservience to the arrogance of science."[38] Blavatsky herself was occasionally quite hostile to contemporary science, though this was due less to a fundamental disagreement with its claims than to her rejection of the materialistic reductionism that often accompanied these claims. For Blavatsky, as for many metaphysical thinkers of her time, science was only beginning to glean the universal truths that esoteric philosophies had uncovered long ago. Thus, while she was suspicious of the authenticity of India's vast population of Yogis, she did not dispute the reality of the phenomena they were reputed to manifest. On this account, her reasoning appealed in no small part to scientific thought, as she wrote:

> Until gravitation is understood to be simply magnetic attraction and repulsion, and the part played by magnetism itself in the endless correlations

of forces in the ether of space—that "hypothetical medium," as Webster terms it, I maintain that it is neither fair nor wise to deny the levitation of either fakir or table. Bodies oppositely electrified attract each other; similarly electrified, repulse each other. Admit, therefore, that any body having weight, whether man or inanimate object, can by any cause whatever, external or internal, be given the same polarity as the spot on which it stands, and what is to prevent its rising?[39]

This passage represents perhaps the most particular rationalization of supernatural phenomena that we find in Blavatsky's writings. This is not to say that Blavatsky was unconcerned with metaphysics but only that rationalizing those metaphysics on the level of gross materiality was near the bottom rung of her priorities. She took for granted the notion of electromagnetism and its ethereal substratum, and went the extra step—which was not an unreasonable one, given that the unity of all forces had been proposed by minds far more scientifically inclined than her own—of declaring them to be identical to the operations of gravitation. Thus, she considered the levitating Yogis (or fakirs) of India were just as scientifically feasible as the tipping tables of Victorian parlors, both being totally accounted for by the magnetic manipulation of a universal force flowing through the ether that modern scientific experimentation was only just beginning to uncover.

Rather than the gross mechanics of supernatural phenomena, which were after all rather mundane, Blavatsky was far more interested in the higher planes of subtle embodiment and the levels of spiritual evolution to which these corresponded. To this end she yoked Swedenborgian notions of the human spirit progressing though successively higher celestial spheres on its path to perfection with Indian cosmologies and a modified theory of reincarnation. This was instrumental in Theosophy's claim to universality in that the Mahatma was understood in this context not as a special class of being specific to a given tradition, but rather as an advanced adept of any background who had mastered the occult sciences and ascended to a superhuman evolutionary state. More precisely, the Mahatma was "a personage, who, by special training and education, has evolved those higher faculties and has attained that spiritual knowledge, which ordinary humanity will acquire after passing through numberless series of re-incarnations during the process of cosmic evolution."[40] Superhumanity was thus the birthright of all of humanity; the Mahatmas were simply a bit ahead of the game.

According to Blavatsky, the subtle embodiment of a genuine Mahatma significantly transcends the etheric or "astral" level of reality on which supernatural phenomena occur. The latter term reflects a Neo-Platonic concept adopted by

Blavatsky from the work of Levi and his notion of the astral light, which was similar in nature to contemporary theories of ether and other subtle media. The schemas of subtle materiality and embodiment introduced by Blavatsky and elaborated on by later Theosophists are ascribed a pivotal role in the Indian frameworks that they adapted to their purposes. It is the ether, however, that, despite being only the lowest of these subtle spheres, is responsible for the observable phenomena manifested by Mahatmas, Yogis, aspiring adepts, and indeed Blavatsky herself.

Interestingly, though Blavatsky remained always in close communion with the Mahatmas, she never attributed any such status to herself. She was, however, quite fond of manifesting all sorts of supernatural phenomena dating back to her days as an extraordinary Spiritualist medium. Strains of music would spontaneously flow through the air, letters would tumble from the ceiling, and lost artifacts would mysteriously reappear. Many of these phenomena were ultimately proven to be fraudulent in the course of the infamous Coulomb scandal and a subsequent report delivered to the British Society for Psychical Research (SPR) by Richard Hodgson.

In 1884 the SPR launched a preliminary investigation into the marvelous phenomena claimed by the Theosophical Society, resulting in a provisional report that fraud was undoubtedly present but that there was good cause to believe that at least some of the phenomena may have been genuine. Shortly thereafter Emma Coulomb, a staff member at the Society's Adyar headquarters, leveled a series of accusations against the reality of Blavatsky's phenomena, ranging from claiming that the Mahatma letters were produced by Blavatsky herself to attributing nocturnal sightings of the Mahatmas to the creative use of a turbaned dummy. The final SPR report, issued following Hodgson's investigation of the phenomena in India, concluded that all of the phenomena could be reasonably attributed either to fraud by Blavatsky or hallucination and "unconscious misrepresentation" by the witnesses and ended with the famous sentence that would come to represent Blavatsky's legacy:

> For our own part, we regard her neither as the mouthpiece of hidden seers, nor as a mere vulgar adventuress; we think that she has achieved a title to permanent remembrance as one of the most accomplished, ingenious, and interesting imposters in history.[41]

It has never been determined, however, to what extent Blavatsky's phenomena were a result of intentional deception on her part. Robert Ellwood has read her as a charismatic mystagogue who embodies "qualities not only of the paradigmatic shaman and magus, but also of the trickster and 'ritual clown.'"[42] Blavatsky herself continued to exhibit a highly ambiguous attitude about her phenomena even after the damning SPR report, sometimes wholeheartedly upholding them, while at other times cynically threatening to disavow them. The trickster archetype may fit her personality best, making her quite at home among the Yogis, if not the Mahatmas, whose mysteries were titillating the Western imagination of her day. Indeed, though her corpulent female frame defied both the contemporary and modern images of such a figure, she might be cautiously regarded as the first of the Western Yogis.

Vivekananda and the Scientific Rehabilitation of the Yogi

For the purposes of this study, of far greater importance than the admittedly unique person of Blavatsky or her phenomena is the metaphysical framework upon which those phenomena relied. This framework would survive the effects of the SPR report and would be elaborated on and propagated by Theosophists and Theosophical sympathizers of both Western and Indian backgrounds. In India, as in America, Theosophy has persisted as an influential, albeit not demographically significant, tradition. Its membership figures, even if they could be effectively documented,[43] reflect rather little of its actual impact, which is far more diffuse in nature. For instance, Yogananda's guru, Sri Yukteswar, was an honorary member of the Theosophical Society despite exhibiting no notable Theosophical inclinations or influence in any of his known work. On the other hand, his contemporary, Vivekananda, to whom we will now turn, evidences the opposite tendency despite his vehement opposition to any association with the Theosophical Society.

Although the influence of Theosophy on Indian metaphysical thought can hardly be understated, it was certainly not the only wellspring of Western esotericism to make its contribution to the Bengali Renaissance. Adding to David Kopf's work on British Orientalism and the modernization of Hinduism as effected by the Brahmo Samāj, Elizabeth De Michelis argues for the already existing prevalence of Western esotericism within Brahmo Samāj ideology. Specifically, she points to the established presence of Freemasonry as well as what she considers to be pseudo-esoteric elements of Unitarianism and the ways in which these influences contributed to an occultization of Neo-Vedāntin thought, most evident in Keshub Chandra Sen's "New Dispensation" (Nabo Bidhan) of the Brahmo Samāj.[44] De Michelis characterizes Sen as "chronologically and ideologically positioned between [Debendranath] Tagore's Neo-Vedāntic Romanticism and Vivekananda's Neo-Vedāntic occultism."[45] Certainly there are seeds of both Tagore's and Sen's iterations of the universalistic "scientific religion" in Vivekananda's work. However, what De Michelis identifies as his "occultism" is actually more indebted to Theosophical metaphysics than to any strictly Neo-Vedāntin elaboration.

Indeed, from a semantic standpoint, "occultism" may be the wrong term for Vivekananda's ideology. He goes so far as to attribute the degeneration of yoga—"one of the grandest of sciences"—to a progressive occultization, claiming that "Mystery-mongering weakens the human brain. . . . Thus Yoga fell into the hands of a few persons who made it a secret, instead of letting the full blaze of daylight and reason fall upon it. They did so that they might have the powers to themselves."[46] In Vivekananda's view, occultism leads directly to superstition, perversion of the truth, and above all denigration of India's spiritual capital. It is perhaps in connection with this reasoning that the influence of Theosophy on Vivekananda's work has been largely overlooked.

By the time that Vivekananda became a major player on the international scene, Blavatsky had passed on and Annie Besant, not Madame Blavatsky and her phenomena, had become the effective face of Theosophy. Due to a potent mix of nationalistic sentiment and no small amount of bad blood, stemming from the cold treatment that he had received from Theosophy's representatives at the World Parliament of Religions in 1893 when he refused to join their Society, Vivekananda was famously unaffectionate toward Theosophy. He maintained:

> This Indian grafting of American Spiritualism—with only a few Sanskrit words taking the place of spiritualistic jargon—Mahâtmâ missiles taking the place of ghostly raps and taps, and Mahatmic inspiration that of obsession by ghosts. . . . the Hindus have enough of religious teaching and teachers amidst themselves even in this Kali Yuga, and they do not stand in need of dead ghosts of Russians and Americans.
>
> . . .
>
> The importation in the case of religion should be mostly on the side of the West, we are sure, and our work has been all along in that line. The only help the religion of the Hindus got from the Theosophists in the West was not a ready field, but years of uphill work, necessitated by Theosophical sleight-of-hand methods. The writer ought to have known that the Theosophists wanted to crawl into the heart of Western Society, catching on to the skirts of scholars like Max Müller and poets like Edwin Arnold, all the same denouncing these very men and posing as the only receptacles of universal wisdom. And one heaves a sigh of relief that this wonderful wisdom is kept a secret. Indian thought, charlatanry, and mango-growing fakirism had all become identified in the minds of educated people in the West, and this was all the help rendered to Hindu religion by the Theosophists.[47]

Vivekananda thus had little patience for the occult and the ostentatious displays of the supranormal. His diagnosis of Theosophy's profound Spiritualist roots is, of course, accurate, though ideologically the Mahatmas are perhaps more closely related to the Adepts of Rosicrucianism than they are to the parlor spooks of Spiritualism. It is clear that Vivekananda has no excess of respect for Blavatsky's phenomena, which he associates with other elements of a popular Yogi's unseemly reputation—that is, "charlatanry" and "mango-growing fakirism." The latter refers to the popular street magic trick, mentioned earlier, that appears in the descriptions of the earliest European travelers in which a mango tree "magically" blossoms from a seed before the very eyes of the audience. It is significant that in Vivekananda's critique he ascribes this trick to the originally Islamic fakir, not the (Hindu) Yogi. In fact, *Raja Yoga* might be read as Vivekananda's attempt to rehabilitate the persona of the Yogi—though this is not his explicit concern—by strategically (re)defining yoga in modern and scientific terms.

Vivekananda, while not denying the reality of yogic superpowers, famously rejected their usefulness in matters of spiritual advancement. Nevertheless, affirming the power of the Yogi is essential to his argument regarding the universal significance of the practice and, more important, the philosophy of yoga. Establishing yoga as a science is fundamental to the thrust of Vivekananda's work, and it is precisely here that the elements that De Michelis has identified with his esoteric *Naturphilosophie*—namely the "Prāṇa Model"—come into play. As De Michelis has observed, Vivekananda's cosmology represents an odd departure from traditional Sāṃkhyan and even Vedāntin notions of cosmogonic emanationalism. Rather than relying on the commonly accepted cosmic substratum of *prakṛti* and its composite *guṇa*s, Vivekananda identifies two primary universal principles: *prāṇa* and *ākāśa*. He proceeds to describe their relationship in *Raja Yoga* as follows:

> By what power is this Akasha manufactured into this universe? By the power of Prana. Just as Akasha is the infinite, omnipresent material of this universe, so is this Prana the infinite, omnipresent manifesting power of this universe. At the beginning and at the end of a cycle everything becomes Akasha, and all the forces that are in the universe resolve back into the Prana; in the next cycle, out of this Prana is evolved everything that we call energy, everything that we call force.[48]

As others have noted,[49] Vivekananda was not a remarkably systematic writer. Even more significantly, he was not a metaphysician in the primary sense. Nevertheless, this schema is carried through the entirety of his collected works and therefore clearly constitutes a coherent metaphysical vision. Other sections of the same text indicate that Vivekananda is aware of Sāṃkhyan metaphysics, the role of *ākāśa*, and the primordial status of *prakṛti*. It is true that *ākāśa* might traditionally be seen as the origin of the material cosmos. According to Sāṃkhya, it is the first and most subtle of the five *mahābhūtas* (gross elements) and thus gives rise to the four subsequent forms of matter, and this position is also articulated in certain Upaniṣadic and Vedāntin passages that name *ākāśa* as the source of gross materiality. However, Vivekananda claims much more than this. In his conception, *ākāśa* becomes identical with *mūlaprakṛti*, the primordial matter to which all creation reverts at the time of cosmic dissolution. This conception is not generally substantiated by Indian sources.

Whence, then, this preoccupation with "Akasha"? It should be noted that, for Vivekananda, *ākāśa* is directly equivalent to the Western notion of ether, both in its classical and modern scientific form. This is not in itself surprising or overly interesting in that "ether" had previously been established as a common translation for "*ākāśa*" by Indologists and the two terms had also been identified in a multitude of Theosophical writings. However, it is only in the Theosophical texts that this identification is understood to imply a particular cosmogonic role. Indeed, Vivekananda's otherwise odd conception of *ākāśa*'s role as primordial matter becomes much clearer when one considers the following passage from Blavatsky's *Isis Unveiled*:

> The modern Ether; not such as is recognized by our scientists, but such as it was known to the ancient philosophers, long before the time of Moses; Ether, with all its mysterious and occult properties, containing in itself the germs of universal creation. . . . Electricity, magnetism, heat, light, and chemical action are so little understood even now that fresh acts are constantly widening the range of our knowledge. Who knows where ends the power of this protean giant—Ether; or whence its mysterious origin?— Who, we mean, that denies the spirit that works in it and evolves out of it all visible forms?[50]

Given Vivekananda's general lack of respect for Theosophy, it is unlikely that he adopted this notion directly from Blavatsky. However, Theosophy had by this time become so diffuse in Indian intellectual circles that it is not unlikely that he might have picked it up from a more loosely affiliated source. Vivekananda's awareness of more traditional Indian cosmologies, especially with respect to notions of subtle embodiment, is evident and his appeal to them unavoidable when he is faced with the task of explaining the states of yogic meditation. However, it is difficult to reconcile such explanations with his references to the *ākāśa/prāṇa* model of materiality.[51] We are thus presented with an interesting turn of events: Blavatsky, who was so fond of occultism that she eventually caused a rift in the Theosophical

Society so that she might start her own "esoteric section," and Vivekananda, who held nothing but disdain for occultism and Theosophy, both made use of the same "occult" scientific concept to justify a cosmos in which supranormal phenomena could take place.

The Unlikely Metaphysical Duo: Vivekananda and Tesla

It is a common tendency among scholars of Vivekananda's writings to dismiss his ambitions of scientific legitimacy. Scholars such as De Michelis characterize his work as an idealistic *Naturphilosophie* of principles that "rather than obeying the laws of Newtonian physics, operate along the lines of more arcane associations between microcosm and macrocosm."[52] With respect to Vivekananda's conviction that Vedānta represented the singular scripture whose teachings could be brought into "entire harmony" with modern science, Carl Jackson maintains that "such assertions must have seemed startling and even absurd to contemporary Western observers."[53] Leaving aside momentarily the fact that Newton essentially created the modern concept of ether while speculating that it might serve as the origin of all natural phenomena, such characterizations are simply not reflective of contemporary scientific thought. In an essay on the nature of ether, Vivekananda links the classic Greek element to the Hindu *ākāśa* as an example of ancient attempts to establish the unity of all physical phenomena, after which he provides a brief but rather thorough summary of modern developments in Western science, beginning with Newton and tracing notable theoretical and experimental landmarks, with the accuracy of a physics textbook. The aim: to find a corollary to *ākāśa* as a universal substratum of matter in contemporary theories of the luminiferous ether.[54]

Toward the end of his sojourn in the United States, Vivekananda was in contact the Nikola Tesla, indicating in a personal letter that "Mr. Tesla thinks he can demonstrate mathematically that force and matter are reducible to potential energy. I am to go and see him next week, to get this new mathematical demonstration."[55] Unfortunately, the demonstration never materialized, though there is evidence that the meeting did in fact occur. Moreover, Tesla's own writings indicate that he was quite in agreement with the spirit of Vivekananda's metaphysics and went so far as to adopt the language of *prāṇa* and *ākāśa* to describe his theories.

As we have seen in the previous chapter, especially with regards to the Yogi's stage magic, the discrediting of paranormal phenomena grew into something of a cottage industry toward the end of the nineteenth century. However, for every scientifically minded detractor who decried the nonsense of parlor séances, there was an equally committed scientist who sought to demonstrate that such phenomena were not only real but thoroughly supported by the laws of physics.[56] Furthermore, "ether metaphysics"[57] were being employed by several European physicists in ways that would strike the modern reader as no less startling and absurd to the modern reader than any claims made by Vivekananda. For instance, there is good reason to believe that the Theosophical concept of the Akashic Record, mentioned at the outset of this chapter as a cosmic repository of all human knowledge, emerged not out of ancient Indian arcana but out of the speculations of contemporary physicists. Scottish physicists Balfour Stewart and Peter Guthrie Tate propose in their anonymously published *The Unseen Universe* (1875) that "what we generally call ether may be not a mere medium, but a medium *plus* the invisible order of things, so that when the motions of the visible universe are transferred into the ether, part of them are conveyed as a bridge into the invisible universe, and are there made use of and stored up."[58] They assert that ether is thus a carrier of dissipating cosmic energies that results in "an arrangement in virtue of which our universe keeps up a memory of the past" such that "continual photographs of all occurrences are thus produced and retained"[59] and indeed "produces a material organ of memory."[60]

Tesla's own legacy, which is now enjoying somewhat of a renaissance in popular culture, was largely forgotten following his death despite the fact that he left behind nearly 300 patents. For instance, though he made many crucial advances in the field of electrical engineering, it is Edison who is remembered as the father of the electric age because, as Tesla's modern editor Samantha Hunt put it, "he gave people something to dance to [with his marketing of the phonograph] while Tesla, with talk of death-rays, lightning bolts, and extraterrestrials, gave a war-weary nation the creeps."[61] His reputation as a fanciful futurist whose aspirations included free energy and the aforementioned death-ray (which was a "teleforce" weapon that Tesla hoped would bring about world peace) notwithstanding, Tesla was generally far less interested in psychic phenomena than some of his contemporaries. In fact, he recounts that he was once approached by "a body of engineers from the Ford Motor Company" who, rather than being interested in his turbines, informed him much to his dismay: "We have formed a psychological society for the investigation of psychic phenomena and we want you to join us in this undertaking."[62] Tesla declined.

Thus, despite Tesla being a bit of an oddball, his inclination toward fanciful flights into the paranormal should not be overstated. Consequently, when Tesla publicly claimed that "to create and annihilate material substance, cause it to aggregate in forms according to his desire, would be the supreme manifestation of Man's mind,"[63] we might take it as legitimate evidence that Vivekananda's ideas may not have been as far from the mainstream of "rational" scientific thought as some have come to believe. What did differentiate Tesla from his contemporaries was his adoption of Indian terminology, though that too would soon come into vogue among the fathers of quantum mechanics as they struggled to explain the theory's problematic blurring of the subject-object relationship. The preceding statement originates from Tesla's "Man's Greatest Achievement," a short essay first delivered as an address in 1908 and subsequently reprinted in several newspapers across the nation over the next few decades. The most striking section of this essay is worth quoting here in its entirety:

> Long ago he [man] recognized that all perceptible matter comes from a primary substance, or a tenuity beyond conception, filling all space, the Akasha or luminiferous ether, which is acted upon by the life-giving Prana or Creative Force, calling into existence, in never ending cycles, all things and phenomena.
>
> The primary substance, thrown into infinitesimal whirls of prodigious velocity, becomes gross matter; the force subsiding, the motion ceases and matter disappears, reverting to the primary substance.
>
> Can man control this grandest, most awe-inspiring of all processes in nature? Can he harness her inexhaustible energies to perform all their functions at his bidding, more still—cause them to operate simply by the force of his will?
>
> If he could do this, he would have powers almost unlimited and super-natural. At his command, with but a slight effort on his part, old worlds would disappear and new ones of his planning would spring into being.
>
> He could fix, solidify and preserve the ethereal shapes of his imagin-ing, the fleeting visions of his dreams. He could express all the creations of his mind on any scale, in forms concrete and imperishable. He could alter the size of this planet, control its seasons, guide it along any path he might choose through the depths of the Universe.
>
> He could make planets to collide and produce his suns and stars, his heat and light. He could originate and develop life in all its infinite forms.[64]

What Tesla describes is nothing short of the powers of the Yogi as presented by Vivekananda, generalized into "man" writ-large. Not coincidentally, his prose is strikingly similar in tone and magnitude to Vivekananda's own words in *Raja Yoga*:

> Suppose, for instance, a man understood the Prana perfectly, and could control it, what power on earth would not be his? He would be able to move the sun and stars out of their places, to control everything in the

universe, from the atoms to the biggest suns, because he would control
the Prana. This is the end and aim of Pranayama. When the Yogi becomes
perfect, there will be nothing in nature not under his control. If he orders
the gods or the souls of the departed to come, they will come at his bidding. All the forces of nature will obey him as slaves. When the ignorant
see these powers of the Yogi, they call them the miracles.

The Yogis say that behind this particular manifestation there is a gener-
alisation. Behind all particular ideas stands a generalised, an abstract principle; grasp it, and you have grasped everything. The Yogi who has done
this gains perfection; no longer is he under any power. He becomes almost
almighty, almost all-knowing.[65]

Directly following this excerpt, Vivekananda acknowledges that Yogis are not
the only ones who have attempted to access this power. He explicitly includes
in this category the varieties of American metaphysical practitioners—mind-
healers, faith-healers, Spiritualists, Christian Scientists, and hypnotists—in whose
company he is likely to have circulated during his time in the United States. In a
universalizing move, Vivekananda argues that yogic superpowers in all their manifestations, which represent a generic attempt to control material nature, rely on a
manipulation of the flow of *prāṇa* through the substratum of *ākāśa*.

Prāṇa and *ākāśa* are converted by Vivekananda into scientific language as
energy and matter. In his perspective, *Prāṇāyāma* therefore relies on a control
of electrical (or nerve) currents as they flow through the material of the body,
which is considered identical to and coextensive with the material of the universe.
It is important to remember that Vivekananda never received formal initiation
into any traditional *sādhana*, or ritual lineage. He therefore spends little time
expounding on the details of yogic practice, and his teachings are generally limited to deep breathing and basic meditation exercises. Nevertheless, in the coupling of breath control and will, he finds all the necessary elements to substantiate
the mechanics of his yogic science:

> In the first place, from rhythmical breathing comes a tendency of all the mol-
> ecules in the body to move in the same direction. When mind changes into
> will, the nerve currents change into a motion similar to electricity, because
> the nerves have been proved to show polarity under the action of electric cur-
> rents. This shows that when the will is transformed into the nerve currents, it
> is changed into something like electricity. When all the motions of the body
> have become perfectly rhythmical, the body has, as it were, become a gigantic
> battery of will. This tremendous will is exactly what the Yogi wants.[66]

Thus, in Vivekananda's perspective, through perfectly scientific methods the Yogi becomes a superman capable to manipulating all forms of matter. *Prāṇa* is defined as force in its most fundamental sense, being responsible for the manifestation of electricity, magnetism, and the nerve force that catalyzes all forms of movement in the body and mind.

For the Yogi who has realized the unity of all matter, the movement does not have to stop there. By tapping into the universal etheric substance, the Yogi can manipulate any manifestation of it that he chooses:

> Similarly, we can send electricity to any part of the world, but we have to send it by means of wires. Nature can send a vast mass of electricity without any wires at all. Why cannot we do the same? We can send mental electricity. What we call mind is very much the same as electricity. It is clear that this nerve fluid has some amount of electricity, because it is polarised, and it answers all electrical directions. We can only send our electricity through these nerve channels. Why not send the mental electricity without this aid? The Yogis say it is perfectly possible and practicable, and that when you can do that, you will work all over the universe. You will be able to work with any body anywhere, without the help of the nervous system.[67]

This scientization of yoga, and by extension of the Yogi, accomplishes two things. First, it brings Western rationalist legitimacy to the Yogi, who had previously been seen as a figure veiled in superstition and mystical exoticism. Second, it serves to universalize the status of the Yogi and the accessibility of his power.

Blavatsky had paved the way for this move by populating her Theosophical narrative with a non-sectarian pantheon of Mahatmas. However, whereas the Mahatmas are already perfected beings whose methods were accessible only by way of the occult, the Yogi is a human figure whose ascent to superhuman status is openly framed in terms of a series of psycho-somatic exercises. Moreover, this methodology relies on analogies to empirically verifiable processes such as electromagnetism and human anatomy. The Yogi simply has to manipulate these natural forces by applying his energized will to the all-pervading etheric medium of conductivity—a notion that was already quite familiar to Vivekananda's Western audiences from the relatively recent heyday of Mesmerism.

Ether and Light in the Quantum Age

Vivekananda's—and Tesla's—assertions are all the more interesting because they were written in a time of crisis within the scientific study of ether. By the time that both men made their claims about the unity of all material manifestation, the Michelson-Morley experiments of 1887 had already cast severe doubt upon the accepted notion of the luminiferous ether. The concept had certainly not been abandoned, especially given that no other scientific explanation for the propagation of light existed, but it was clear that a new theory was needed.

Tesla wrote "Man's Greatest Achievement" only three years after Albert Einstein first proposed his special theory of relativity in 1905. In doing so, Einstein accomplished a version of what Tesla had promised Vivekananda a decade prior, proving the equivalence of mass and energy $(E = mc^2)$ and eliminating the need for the ether as a universal frame of reference to explain electrodynamics. Einstein also belonged to a cohort of quantum physicists who observed that light can in fact be understood as particles that exhibit a wave-like nature—the beginning of modern quantum mechanics—thereby effectively eliminating the requirement of a medium for the propagation of electromagnetic waves. By 1946, when Yogananda published his *Autobiography*, it was no longer scientifically tenable to refer to a material ether. This only meant, however, that the cypher of subtle materiality represented by ether moved yet another step farther from material reality as we see it. Indeed, as late as 1920 Einstein himself insisted in his famous Leyden address that "there is a weighty argument to be adduced in favour of the Aether hypothesis" since "to deny the Aether is ultimately to assume that empty space has no physical qualities whatever," and finally concluded that "according to the General Theory of Relativity, space without Aether is unthinkable."[68] Of course, this new ether had few of the same characteristics as its predecessor, yet the general concept persisted. Eventually, however, theories of electromagnetism relying on the dual nature of light radiation and the role of its speed as a universal constant ushered in a new era of metaphysical theorizing that would attempt to establish light, rather than its now defunct medium, as the raw material of all creation.

In this new age of electromagnetic theory, the spiritual telegraph of the medium became the mental radio of the channel. The language of energy and light as representative of the spiritual is overwhelmingly characteristic of New Age metaphysics.[69] Here we begin to see a transition in registers. Although the first wireless radio transmissions were achieved in the late 1890s, it was not until the early 1920s that radio broadcasting truly entered the public sphere. With the advent of technology capable of carrying the human voice over long distances by invisible but incontestably real and scientific means, energetic transmission found a new foothold in metaphysical thought. Albanese traces the language of channeling to the technological shamanist of the UFO contactee movement of the 1950s,[70] but the basic language of mind as radio begins well before this.

Upton Sinclair's *Mental Radio*, published in 1930, painstakingly catalogs his wife's experiments and relative success with the practice of telepathy. Sinclair, who generally abstained from either scientific or metaphysical speculation as to the basis of his wife's mental powers nevertheless noted: "The human brain is a storage battery, capable of sending impulses over the nerves. Why may it not be capable of sending impulses by means of some other medium, known or unknown? Why may there not be such a thing as brain radio?"[71] The analogy to nerve impulses should be familiar as it takes us directly back to Vivekananda's work—which, it must be noted, Sinclair might well have been familiar with—however, the difference is that Sinclair's "brain radio" existed in a time when remote transmission of electric impulse was no longer science fiction but quotidian reality. While the general population hardly knew *how* the voice of a person speaking from forty miles away was filtering into devices in their parlors, no one could deny that this seemingly magical phenomenon was happening. The electromagnetic waves of radio transmissions thus became the perfect analogy for telepathic and even telekinetic phenomena. The concurrent advent of motion picture technology added yet another layer. Although the old material aspects of ether were slowly fading from metaphysical discourse, they were only making room for a new more dynamic form of subtle materiality—a materiality that was hardly material at all but, like light, largely energetic.

Taking this into account, one can approach Yogananda's work as a moment in the transition between these two registers. An examination of his *Autobiography*, which is both the latest and the most thorough representation of his metaphysics, yields a conflicting vision. On the one hand, the language of ether is fairly prominent, not only as a figurative descriptor of subtle materiality, but in references to actual phenomena. When objects or people materialize or dematerialize, they do so from and into the ether. On the other hand, he makes use of the language of "mental radio," referring to his guru, Sri Yukteswar, not only as a "perfect human radio" but also as a "human broadcasting station" capable of transmitting his thoughts and will over great distances to effect desired phenomena.[72]

Indeed, when Yogananda evoked the language of magnetism, it would manifest as a kind of vibrational current, which he would at times describe as being analogous to a subtle form of electricity. Explicitly building on Mesmer's animal magnetism, he maintained that these energies were emitted by every body but became especially perceptible when coupled with conscious will. However, such magnetic vibrations were not quite as value-neutral as common notions of electricity. They could be good or bad and can constitute a kind of mana, which Yogananda illustrated with the common example of why people like to shake hands with the famous. Furthermore, he disclosed that it was possible to "steal" magnetism (good vibrations) from saints simply by being in their presence. For this specific reason, Yogananda used to perform daily "broadcasts" of his vibrations between the hours of seven and eleven in the morning and encouraged his devotees to "tune in."[73]

In this context, Yogananda relies on a the older model of ether as a medium of electromagnetic propagation when he specifies that "in telepathy the fine vibrations of thoughts in one person's mind are transmitted through the subtle vibrations of astral ether and then through the grosser earthly ether, creating electrical waves which, in turn, translate themselves into thought waves in the mind of the other person."[74] Here the dual terminology of the "astral ether" is consistent with his larger claims regarding the nature of subtle materiality. However, the notion of the "grosser earthly ether" appears to be in direct contradiction to statements such as:

> Even the hypothetical ether, held as the interplanetary medium of light in the undulatory theory, can be discarded on the Einsteinian grounds that the geometrical properties of space render the theory of ether unnecessary. Under either hypothesis, light remains the most subtle, the freest from material dependence, of any natural manifestation.[75]

Generally speaking, for Yogananda, light itself, rather than the "gross" material ether, becomes the subtlest aspect of materiality. Thus, when the term "ether" appears in his work, it is generally describing something slightly different than the luminiferous ether referred to by his predecessors. The notion of light as a unique universal constant becomes the ground of subtle materiality. Due to its dual nature as both a particle (gross matter) and a wave (energy), light becomes identified with the "astral ether" insofar as it serves as the bridge between matter and spirit.

The Sanskrit *akāśa* is markedly absent from Yogananda's language, though this may be mostly due to his preference for English terminology. On the few occasions that the term appears in his work, he identifies it with ether as well as with the Theosophical concept of the Akashic Records, which he defines as "audible sounds vibrating from the ether."[76] Moreover, even though ether itself does make a number of appearances, Yogananda generally prefers to rely on a familiar Theosophical synonym—the "astral." As previously noted, the latter term derives from Neo-Platonism and its Hermetic and European occult evolutes. However, it is popularized by Theosophy as equivalent to the aspects of subtle materiality that are commonly referred to as "astral body" and "astral plane," and thus becomes a common staple of metaphysical parlance. In Yogananda's case, however, it is likely that the term "astral" is preferred over its common synonym, "ether," largely due to its even stronger light-based connotations.

The primary tenet of Yogananda's metaphysics thus rests on the claim that "the essence of all objects is light"[77] and the visible material cosmos therefore operates as a tangible holographic image. This results in a fairly thorough reinterpretation of traditional Sāṃkhyan metaphysics brought into agreement with the popular scientific understandings of Yogananda's time. "Popular" is a crucial term here because, despite his preoccupation with light, Yogananda appears to be unaware of the existence of photons, the quanta of light and all other forms of electromagnetic radiation that had been acknowledged by the scientific community some twenty years prior to the *Autobiography*'s publication in 1946. Consequently, for Yogananda there are protons, there are electrons, and then there are "lifetrons." More specifically, all sensory stimuli result from the vibrations of protons and electrons, which are in turn regulated by lifetrons or "subtle life forces or finer-than-atomic energies intelligently charged with the five distinctive sensory idea substances."[78] Lifetrons are essentially *prāṇa*. Indeed, Yogananda explicitly equates the two terms but almost uniformly chooses to employ his translation in place of the original Sanskrit, giving his metaphysical speculations a distinctly scientific tone. To Yogananda's credit, unlike Vivekananda, he manages to fully integrate his scientific vision into the subject-based emanation theory that underlies traditional Indian Sāṃkyan and Vedāntin cosmologies. We will turn to a closer examination of his schema of subtle embodiment in chapter 5. In the present context, it is enough to say that Yogananda's vision of materiality rests on a kind of quantum monism.

Whereas Vivekananda relied on a *prāṇa/ākāśa* duality—electromagnetic energy and its medium, the ether—to explain natural phenomena, Yogananda is able to reduce the entirety of matter into a single substratum of light. Yogananda posits an astral universe composed of lifetrons underlying all gross matter. *Prāṇa* then becomes both matter and energy—insofar as matter is simply "congealed" energy—which are both rendered as light. This is where Yogananda's explanations require a bit of interpretation. Although Yogananda never explicitly states that lifetrons are particles of light, this appears to be the only logical conclusion. Being unaware of the photon as a distinct quantum particle, Yogananda seems to extrapolate from Einstein's mass-energy equivalence that if the speed of light is the universal constant that makes this equivalence possible, then it must mean that all mass as well as all energy is ultimately reducible to light. This effectively allows him to create a new universal substratum—a new ether of sorts—now manifesting as an underlying astral universe composed of a "throbbing stream of lifetrons."[79]

Asserting this quantum monism opens up a whole new vista of possibilities for explaining the most "magical" of yogic superpowers. Relying on a formulation of the "magnification" of the yogic body, Yogananda asserts that "only a material body whose mass is infinite could equal the velocity of light."[80] Yogis, having realized their cosubstantiality with the entirety of the energetic cosmos, rely on exactly this principle:

> Masters who are able to materialize and dematerialize their bodies and other objects, and to move with the velocity of light, and to utilize the creative light rays in bringing into instant visibility any physical manifestation, have fulfilled the lawful condition: their mass is infinite.[81]

In reality, this is somewhat of a misreading of Einstein's actual theory, to which Yogananda appeals to substantiate this conclusion. Technically speaking, it is not so much that only a body of infinite mass is capable of achieving the speed of light but that any massive body would become infinitely massive as it approaches light speed. Consequently, massive bodies are not generally capable of such a feat because they would require an infinite amount of force (or energy) to accelerate their infinite mass to reach light speed. From a modern scientific perspective, Yogananda might have gained more traction by claiming that Yogis are capable of attaining light speeds by becoming massless, as photons are, and thereby appealing to the canonical superpower of *laghimā* (minimization) rather than *mahimā* (magnification).[82]

Regardless of the objective accuracy of Yogananda's physics, however, it remains significant that his justification of yogic power remains fundamentally and intentionally scientific. Indeed, by appealing to a form—albeit an ultimately invented form—of quantum physics, Yogananda is able to more fully integrate traditional Indian thought, modern science, and prevailing Western metaphysical notions of will, mind, and consciousness. The modern Yogi, who has now effectively returned to his traditional mode of light-based apotheosis, is able to manipulate astral quanta of the universe at will:

> A yogi who though perfect meditation has merged his consciousness with the Creator perceives the cosmical essence as light (vibrations of life energy); to him there is no difference between the light rays composing water and the light rays composing land. Free from matter-consciousness, free from the three dimensions of space and the fourth dimension of time, a master transfers his body of light with equal ease over and through the light rays of earth, water, fire, and air.[83]

In tapping into this uniformity of matter, the Yogi's domain becomes limitless. An old concept therefore finds a new, perhaps even more expansive, form. Rather than relying on the crude fluid dynamics of the ether, this new Yogi's body and powers are purely energetic.

In our present context, however, it is worth noting that even as Yogananda places the (realized) Yogi beyond the realm of materiality, even the highest of perfected beings make their appearances through language permeated with the terminology of material science. This is exemplified in following narration of an immortal and fully liberated "avatar":

> There was a sudden flash; we witnessed the instantaneous dechemicaliza-
> tion of the electronic elements of Babaji's body into a spreading vaporous
> light. The God-tuned will power of the master had loosened its grasp of
> the ether atoms held together as his body; forthwith the trillions of tiny
> lifetronic sparks faded into the infinite reservoir.[84]

Even fully perfected Yogis are made of ether atoms.

Yogananda's light-based quantum monism thus marks the shift to a new para-digm. When Rhonda Byrne's *The Secret* (2006)—perhaps the most mainstream example of New Age exoteric esoterica to date—purports to guide its adherents in living their lives "in accordance with the natural laws of the Universe," this language carries no small amount of literal meaning. For Byrne, the most fun-damental cosmic law is the "Law of Attraction"—a phrase first coined in 1906 by New Thought author William Walter Atkinson (1862–1932) in his *Thought Vibration or The Law of Attraction in the Thought World,* but still alive and well in the twenty-first century. In Byrne's view, every human being—not just a per-fected Yogi master, as Yogananda might have claimed—is capable of functioning as a "perfect human radio." After all, if both thoughts and material objects can be broken down into a common substratum of energy, then why should each person not be able to calibrate her thoughts to the proper frequency for attracting the desired object? This is perhaps in part what Yogananda meant when he advertised his lectures with the tagline, "Your Super Powers Revealed!"[85]

3

Here Comes the Yogiman

We're all stories in the end.
—"THE BIG BANG," *Doctor Who*

IN 1948, A seventeen-year-old boy lay bedridden with rheumatoid fever in the small town of Leavittsburg, Ohio. This boy, struck down in the prime of his senior year of high school, was Roy Eugene Davis. He would go on to found the multi-branch Center for Spiritual Awareness, launch the publication of a magazine, and author nine books. In 1948, however, Davis read more books than he wrote:

> I had already read many books that I borrowed from the County Library. Books on psychology and religious movements appealed to me, as did some poems by Alfred Lord Tennyson and the writings of Ralph Waldo Emerson, Henry David Thoreau, and Walt Whitman. I learned about yoga practices while reading Francis Yeats-Brown's *Lives of a Bengal Lancer*, Paul Brunton's *Search in Secret India*, and Theos Bernard's *Hatha Yoga*. I began to practice Hatha Yoga, which I could easily do, and tried to meditate. Alone in my upstairs bedroom, I sometimes sat on the floor in a lotus pos-ture and imagined that I was a spiritually accomplished Himalayan yogi.
>
> While I was confined to bed, I read articles in health-oriented maga-zines that motivated me to choose a vegetarian diet. In one magazine, I saw an advertisement for *Autobiography of a Yogi* by Paramahansa Yogananda, published by Self-Realization Fellowship and ordered a copy by mail. As soon as I received it, I read it, then read it frequently. As I avidly perused the text and looked at the pictures of saints and yogis, I knew that Paramahansa Yogananda was my guru.[1]

Within the year, Davis would travel to the Mt. Washington Center in Los Angeles to meet his guru, an encounter that would begin over sixty years of involvement with Kriya Yoga. Like many of Yogananda's disciples, Davis's first exposure to the Yogi was through his narrative. After the release of Yogananda's *Autobiography* and perhaps even more so after his death, much of the SRF's promotional energy was redirected to disseminating the work.

However, long before Yogananda's story trickled into American homes via his favored method of dissemination—mail-order—and certainly before it was available on the shelves of most bookstores, the Yogi was already making a stir. The *Los Angeles Times* declared in 1932:

> From a standpoint of public interest, the most spectacular swami in Los Angeles is Swami Yogananda, whose headquarters are at Mt. Washington Center, Highland Park. This man, with his long, dark hair and midnight eyes, numbers his followers by the thousands. In his little colony on the hill are scores of men and women who seem devoted to him and his doctrines, and his lectures on Sunday afternoons attract hundreds of persons, some humble and ignorant, others merely curious.[2]

Yogananda's long hair and midnight eyes had already been enchanting—as well as perturbing—American audiences all over the nation for over a decade. It was only a few years after arriving in Boston with hardly a foothold to rely on that he progressed to lecturing before auditoriums and concert halls filled to brimming capacity. His methods for capturing the rapt attention of his audiences varied from feats of physical strength and superhuman abilities to engaging philosophical expositions on the mysteries of mind, matter, and divinity.

The berobed representative of the Maharaja of Kasimbazar of Bengal appears to have navigated the line separating his "demonstrations" from the sideshow curiosities and parlor tricks often associated with his contemporaries in the popular imagination with impressive deftness. Yet it was exactly that touch of mysterious power that drew many of his followers, whose personal memoirs never fail to mention at least a few occasions on which their Master displayed an intuition so uncanny as to be superhuman. For disciples like Roy Davis, Yogananda was the embodiment of the mystical stories of India and the presence of the Yogi himself must surely have compensated for the lack of more colorful displays of levitation and the like, which were more comfortably confined to the imagined world of the holy land itself.

The story of the man who became the Yogi, which this chapter attempts to tell, is nevertheless still a story. Unlike Yogananda's *Autobiography*, which reads something like a Dickensian novel, this story is conflicted and fragmentary. In the former, Yogananda appears as something of a superhuman Oliver Twist—a prototypically pure soul moving along the neat arc of his prescribed progress as he offers us colorful glimpses of countless supporting characters and the myriads of details that make up his world, all presented to the reader to illustrate one intended lesson or another. The latter is messier, less linear, at times more surreal in its swirl of chance meetings, students who came to think they were lions, and Polish Yogis from Cleveland. It is *Oliver Twist* redone by David Lynch. Yet this version of the story is no less constructed in its nature or less mythic in its proportions. It is a play—at times antagonistic—between Yogananda's own narrative as it was lived and enacted by him and the categories and storylines imposed onto it by society, by his followers and his detractors, by the media, and by his blood kin and the family of his monastic order. It consists of legend and history and gossip.

This chapter intentionally avoids any direct reference to the *Autobiography* itself. That is the project of chapter 5. Instead, it draws on biographies and personal memoirs published by Yogananda's disciples, who tend to be rather sympathetic, as well as childhood friends, associates, and members of his Indian lineage, who tend to be less so. It also refers to archival sources including newspaper accounts, printed advertisements, and editorials. Finally, it includes personal accounts by SRF members, current and former, found in the many Internet communities that have sprung up to both exalt and criticize Yogananda.

Perhaps most interesting and occasionally frustrating is the fact that Yogananda was in many ways the first to tell his story, exempting the fragmented documentation provided by contemporary media. His *Autobiography of a Yogi* truly is the Ur-narrative in the sense that nearly all other biographical accounts, published and anecdotal, all criticisms, accusations, praises, and elaborations reference Yogananda's work on at least one occasion. It is as though a reference in the *Autobiography* becomes the stamp of legitimacy required to prove that an event—especially a controversial event—actually transpired.[3] In many ways, then, as much as one may try, it is rarely possible to escape entirely the realm of Yogananda's subjectivity.

It is also for this reason that Yogananda's life provides such an apt case study for examining the life of a Yogi, in whatever conflicting ways the category might be understood. The ensuing pages will demonstrate the ways in which Yogananda followed, sometimes intentionally and other times not, the scripted tropes that defined Yogis—modern and premodern, Indian and Westernized—which we have reviewed in the preceding chapters. After all, as the title of his work suggests, a Yogi is precisely and above all else what Yogananda perceived himself to be.

Himalayan Yogis and Swami Orders, or The Making of a Lineage

It is a truth universally acknowledged that an aspiring Yogi in want of a good fortune must be in possession of a lineage. The story of Yogananda thus inevitably begins with the story of Babaji. Although sources vary on Babaji's precise identity and his status as an *avatāra*, a fully-realized immortal being, or simply an extremely advanced adept, there is unanimous consensus within Yogananda's lineage that Babaji was responsible for the recovery of the teachings of Kriya Yoga and their transmission to Lahiri Mahasaya.

Yogananda reports that Lahiri Mahasaya, whose full birth name was Shyama Charan Lahiri, was born on September 30, 1828, though other sources claim that the exact date is not known but has been conjectured to be in 1829.[4] There are few specific accounts of Lahiri Mahasaya's early life and even fewer of his family background. His father is mentioned as a practitioner of yoga and his mother as a Śaiva devotee, though no extraordinary religious fervor is attributed to either of them by anyone other than Yogananda. In any case, it appears that Lahiri Mahasaya lived a perfectly ordinary life until his encounter with Babaji in 1861. He married, had two sons and two daughters, and had a fruitful if unremarkable career as a clerk for the Military Engineering Department of the British government. At the age of thirty-three, he received a transfer to Ranikhet and it was there, in the midst of the Himalayas, that the fateful meeting with Babaji occurred.

Due to the legendary character of this contact, Lahiri Mahasaya's interactions with Babaji will be more fully discussed in chapter 5. Suffice it to say that after 1861 he is regarded as having received initiation into the lost science of Kriya Yoga and became qualified to initiate others. Having been instructed by Babaji to serve as an example of the ideal Yogi-householder, Lahiri Mahasaya held his government post for another twenty-five years. During this time, it is said that he would initiate one or two people into the *sādhana* as time permitted. It was only after his retirement that he began to gather a significant number of disciples. He died on September 26, 1895, when Yogananda was only two years old; however, both of Yogananda's parents received initiation from him. Lahiri Mahasaya never belonged to any official order nor took any formal vows of renunciation. His authority appears to have rested solely on his initiation by Babaji into Kriya Yoga. On a practical level, his apparent level of education and proficiency in the traditional literary canon likely played a significant role. He produced no original written works in the formal sense, but he did publish twenty-six commentaries on texts ranging from the classical *darśana* schools, to Pāṇini's grammar, to various Upaniṣads and devotional texts, including the poetry of Kabīr, to Abhinavagupta's *Tantrasāra*. The *Bhagavad Gītā* appears to have been a particular favorite and was the principal text read and studied by his circle of devotees. Among the publications of Lahiri Mahasaya's disciples, commentaries on the *Bhagavad Gītā* are definitively the most plentiful.

Of all of Lahiri Mahasaya's biographers, Yogananda is by far the most liberal in attributing manifestations of superpowers to the man. The biography penned by Satyananda, Yogananda's childhood friend and later collaborator, does affirm Yogananda's claim that, following his death, Lahiri Mahasaya was seen by three different disciples in vastly different locations. However, for the most part his biographers limit his superhuman abilities to things like supreme omniscience, kindness, and detachment.[5] It is only in Yogananda's accounts that we see Lahiri Mahasaya performing actions such as levitating, delaying trains, inducing visions, and raising the dead. However, given that Yogananda's only encounter with Lahiri Mahasaya occurred when the former was only an infant, the accounts must have been relayed to him by other disciples. Thus, assuming that Yogananda did not simply invent the stories to embellish his own account, tales of Lahiri Mahasaya's powers as told by his devotees must have been much less modest than the other published accounts would suggest.

As to the historicity of Lahiri Mahasaya's initiation into Kriya Yoga by the immortal Babaji, it is uncertain where biography ends and hagiography begins. Given the breadth and complexity of his published commentaries, it is not unlikely that he might have picked up quite a bit of material simply by means of independent study. However, the details of the Kriya Yoga practice, insofar as they have been made available through the publications of Lahiri Mahasaya's disciples in India, suggest a fairly complex tantric *sādhana*. While it is possible that Lahiri Mahasaya might have elaborated on the metaphysical elements of the practice based on his own knowledge, the method itself must have been taught to him via oral transmission by an actual adept. Given the highly abstruse nature of tantric ritual manuals, it would be nearly impossible for one to acquire anything beyond a basic theoretical understanding of the physical mechanics of the practice. Thus, Babaji, immortal or otherwise, appears to be a necessary character in the saga. Whether Kriya Yoga truly constitutes a lost ancient practice is far more doubtful. No full description of the method is available to non-initiates. However, the existing information points to a form of tantric or, even more likely, *haṭha* yogic *sādhana* based primarily on the practice of *prāṇāyāma*. Among the major elements, or *kriyās*, are relatively familiar practices such as *khecarī mudrā* (the extension of the tongue upwards into the nasal cavity), which, despite being esoteric, were by no means lost prior to the middle of the nineteenth century.[6]

Yogananda's own guru, Sri Yukteswar,[7] was born Priyanath Karar on May 10, 1865, in Serampore. Sri Yukteswar was educated at Serampore Christian Missionary College and spent some time at Calcutta Medical School before family matters forced him to abandon both. He married and had one daughter, working as an accountant for some time. Building on his earlier training, Sri Yukteswar studied naturopathic medicine and was interested in physical culture. A particular obsession of his was astrology, which he firmly considered to be scientific rather than mystical. Indeed, young Sri Yukteswar never did hold much regard for yogic superpowers:

> Whenever he heard about some great yogi and his powers, he would visit him. Naturally, he became curious about all yogis. But Priyanath had the conviction that whatever he heard about the mystic powers of certain yogis was not true. In most cases, he thought these were fantastic stories and rumors spread by devotees who hoped to raise the status, name and fame of their Master. Priyanath commented on several occasions that the exhibition by a yogi of yogic powers "cut his figure short" in society. He said, "It is true that even impossible things are made possible by the grace of the Lord through yogic powers, but it is not wise to speak about these happenings or manifestations without fully understanding their deeper implications. To discuss these things emotionally spoils the atmosphere of seriousness, which results in developing disrespect." Priyanath repeatedly warned that one should not be tempted by this cheap way of gaining popularity. Whenever he heard about the extraordinary feats of some yogis, he decided to test their powers. He would use all types of tests.[8]

These "tests" included things such as hiding under the bed of a Yogi who was purported to levitate at night. The Yogi never did become airborne, and Sri Yukteswar, understandably bored, revealed himself by inquiring from underneath the bed when this feat might finally transpire, at which point his presence was blamed for the deficient quality of the Yogi's *samādhi* that evening.

Aside from his myth-busting fascination with Yogis, in his early years Sri Yukteswar is never described as possessing any extraordinary spiritual thirst. His wife died due to illness, though it is not known in what year. Their only daughter died a few years later, and Sri Yukteswar was left with no living blood relatives, except his granddaughter, who was married soon thereafter, and his mother, with whom he maintained a distant relationship. His introduction to Lahiri Mahasaya appears to have been prompted by sheer curiosity, perhaps the same inclination that had driven him to seek out Yogis in his younger days. Nevertheless, in 1883 he received Kriya Yoga initiation in Benares and acknowledged Lahiri Mahasaya as his guru. Following this event, Sri Yukteswar is said to have traveled widely to study with different masters and adepts. A particularly memorable episode recounted by him involved an observation of a particular "aboriginal Master's" *sādhana* that "required a fullmoon night to practice and spiritually dance in a very secret way."[9] Witnessing a group of male and female disciples gathered to dance the *rāsa līlā*,[10] Sri Yukteswar was profoundly touched by the purity of their devotion and the earnestness of their practice. His own approach, however, was always more philosophical in nature. Drawing on his interactions with tantric, Vaiṣṇava, and Baul practitioners, Sri Yukteswar emphasized the hidden commonality of all paths.[11] This same synthetic project occupied his efforts in the work that Babaji personally charged Sri Yukteswar with to write upon their encounter at the Kumbha Mela festival in 1894: *Kaivalya Darśanam*, or *The Holy Science*, under which title it is now published by the SRF.

Sri Yukteswar converted his two-story Serampore home into an ashram and in 1903 founded a second establishment, the Karar Ashram in Puri. Around this time, Sri Yukteswar, then still Priyanath Karar, received advice that proper initiation into an established monastic order might be beneficial for the propagation of Kriya Yoga and the respectability of his establishments. He consequently made haste to Bodh Gaya, where he was initiated by Swami Krishnadayal into the Giri branch of the Daśanāmi Saṃpradāya. It does not appear that he had any prior relationship with Krishnadayal, and the affiliation thus served primarily as a legitimating function. Nevertheless, Swamis initiated into the Kriya Yoga tradition generally belong to the Giri suborder as a matter of lineage.

The importance of lineage should not be understated. Just as Sri Yukteswar found it advantageous to affiliate himself with a formal tradition in order to secure the reputation of his ashrams, so belonging to a "genuine" order of Swamis must have elevated Yogananda's credibility in the eyes of his American audiences. Every metaphysical teacher claiming the title of "Yogi" would generally have had a legitimating narrative about having studied with Himalayan masters, and even Blavatsky had made use of this device in her day. However, being able to put names and (photographic) faces to this narrative no doubt significantly raised Yogananda's spiritual capital.

The Boy Who Wanted Superpowers

Yogananda, then Mukunda Lal Ghosh, was born on January 5, 1893, in Gorakhpur in the state of Uttar Pradesh. The known details of Yogananda's early childhood are extensively treated in his *Autobiography* and need not be recapitulated here. Yogananda is everywhere described as a highly spiritual child. His fervor to become a Yogi intensified after the death of his mother in 1904 and appears to have received special confirmation when, a year later, his brother conveyed to him a special message regarding his destiny that had been given to his mother by Lahiri Mahasaya when Yogananda was only an infant.[12] His father, Bhagavati Charan Ghosh, a direct disciple of Lahiri Mahasaya, initiated him into the first *kriyā* of the Kriya Yoga *sādhana* in 1906. This was the same year that young Yogananda attempted for the second time to run away to the Himalayas to become a *saṃnyāsin*, only to be retrieved within days by his older brother.

Swami Satyananda, then Manamohan Mazumder, was a childhood friend of Yogananda and accompanied him through many of his early adventures. He later became a close associate in the maintenance of Yogananda's organizations and came extremely close to joining him in America. In addition to these administrative duties, Satyananda became one of Yogananda's chief biographers outside of Yogananda himself. From him we know that, at the age of approximately fourteen or fifteen, Yogananda became interested in visiting graveyards and performing *sādhana* on corpses. Satyananda, who had been prevailed upon by Yogananda to join in these outings on occasion, specifies that strictly speaking no *sādhana* had really taken place but only some *japa* (chanting) and contemplation. Yogananda's brother Sananda Lal Ghosh likewise reports that Yogananda for some time dabbled in tantra. He would often visit the Nimtala charnal grounds, where his mother's body had been cremated, until one time he brought home an imposing red-eyed *sādhu*. The pair would disappear into Yogananda's attic room, where his brother discovered one day a human skull along with two bones resting on a wooden stand. Quite disconcerted, he reported these findings to their father, who warned Yogananda about the potential harm of tantric practice. After this, Ghosh claims, Yogananda ceased his experimentation and would later come to warn others against tantric ritual.[13]

From a young age, Yogananda appears to have been fascinated by the concept of yogic superpowers. This is evident from the extensive cataloging of his visits to various Yogis and the preoccupation with supernatural occurrences that color his *Autobiography*. However, the accounts of his biographers affirm that this was more than a gimmick to titillate the Western imagination. Satyananda reports:

> [Yogananda] was very much attracted to the effects of yogic powers, fruition through willpower, and what could be learned from supernatural accounts and other such things. And at this time, he was also seized by the desire to follow practices that would bring about these powers within himself. He was always firmly convinced in the depths of his being that the instrument of intense power of will in a human being's mind empowered by union with the Divine Infinite Power, or the Divine Power using the instrument of the power of human will, could make the impossible possible.[14]

Once Yogananda, with Satyananda at his side, spent a few days harassing lizards in an attempt to implement of some method that he had reportedly learned from a tantric *sādhaka* in the hope of gaining some superpowers of his own. Eventually the boys were overcome with the spirit of nonviolence and took pity on the poor lizards, who had likely not enjoyed being hung upside down. It is unclear whether the *sādhaka* who recommended this method was the same one who so perturbed Yogananda's brother.

Aspiring *tāntrika* or otherwise, Yogananda definitely had a flair for the supernatural. Satyananda again recounts:

> Direct encounters with ascended beings, the radiant and divine appearances of supernatural power-endowed realized beings, the arrival of the spirit of a dead person in the midst of mesmerized people and speaking with that spirit, and ordinary sightings of ghosts and such were things that he [Yogananda] believed in, and pursued with concentrated means in situations and occasions.[15]

This "pursuit" on Yogananda's part manifested particularly in his experimentation with what might be best identified as a form of Mesmerism. During roughly the same time period as his tantric explorations, Yogananda practiced a form of mental control and at other times engaged in full-blown mediumistic possession.

It is not clear where Yogananda acquired these techniques or whether they were based on native Indian or imported Western practices. Yogis are traditionally quite capable of controlling the minds of others. However, Western Mesmerism was also existent in India at the time.[16] Satyananda, who witnessed Yogananda perform the feat on multiple occasions, refers to it as *sammohan vidya* or hypnotism.[17] Yogananda would induce a trance state in his subjects—usually young boys—through gaze, manual contact, or occasionally by sheer application of will. Satyananda claims that his friend never took any lessons on the subject, implying that this was somewhat of a natural ability. As Yogananda's practice had no apparent ritual complexity, it is possible that he acquired the skill simply from observing others. It is equally likely that he had tutors of whose existence his friend was not aware. Yogananda's younger brother was a favorite subject on which he practiced his exercises of mental power:

> I well remember the first time he [Yogananda] asked my help. Our youngest uncle had lived for some time in our house and had been afflicted with a chronic illness. One day Mejda [Yogananda] called me to his prayer room and asked me to sit in a cross-legged posture facing him. Slowly he passed his hand over my head and body. I felt a soothing, relaxing sensation spread through every cell. We talked for a few minutes about trivial matters, then Mejda asked me about our uncle's health. "Uncle's condition

is most serious," I replied. Then I made a remark out of context: "Someone will call you in a moment."

    Almost immediately a knock on the door interrupted us. Mejda was told that someone was at the front door downstairs and wanted to see him.[18]

Occasionally, Yogananda's sessions with his younger brother took on the more troubling character of spirit-possession:

> Mejda was then experimenting with spiritualism; he used me as a medium to contact departed souls. On one occasion a soul took possession of my passive mind and body, and was unwilling to give up its newly acquired residence. He said that he had been murdered near Talla Bridge and desperately wanted another physical form. He was determined to keep mine![19]

Fortunately, Yogananda was eventually able to exorcise the malicious spirit using an image of Lahiri Mahasaya. With similar mediumistic aid, he was able on at least one occasion to contact his deceased mother in the "astral world."

    If relying on Western terminology, these practices might in a mixed fashion fall under the purview of both Spiritualism—which is the term Ghosh uses—and Mesmerism. The latter is probably more correct, given Yogananda's active presence in the event, especially where it concerns his use of suggestion. However, there is little evidence besides Satyananda's vague but evocative statement regarding Yogananda's interests, cited earlier, to illuminate what he might have actually been exposed to in the way of source material, whether Western or Indian in origin.[20] Eventually, like Yogananda's foray into tantra, these practices would be given up at his father's reprimand. Later, in his *Autobiography*, he would acknowledge the relative effectiveness of hypnotism, especially in medical contexts, but would reject it as a temporary phenomenon having "nothing in common with the miracles performed by men of divine self-realization,"[21] which is at best unethical and at worst damaging to the brain. However, the attribution of some form of hypnotic ability, whether sensationalized, censorious, or glorifying, would follow Yogananda for the majority of his career.

Yogananda's Influences and the Genesis of a Modern Yogi

Although little remains to shed light on some of Yogananda's more esoteric influences, there are some more well-documented sources that played an important role in the early formation of his thought. One important point of interest is

Yogananda's fondness for the famous mystic Ramakrishna, guru to another transnational Yogi. In his teenage years, Yogananda regularly frequented the Kali temple in Dakshineshwar and especially liked to meditate in Ramakrishna's favorite spots on the grounds. Despite the ambivalent attitude that Yogananda would develop toward Ramakrishna's celebrated disciple Vivekananda and his organization, he would always retain a reverential regard for the old mystic. Yogananda used to carry in his pocket a book of advice by Ramakrishna, written by Swami Brahmananda, and was quite enamored of Mahedranath Gupta (Sri "M" or "Master Mahasaya" in Yogananda's *Autobiography*), another prominent disciple of Ramakrishna who was the author of *Sri Ramakrishna Kathamrita* (1905).

Although Vivekananda's path must certainly have served as a model for Yogananda's own ambitions—perhaps all the more so due to the sense of implicit competition that he would later develop—Swami Rama Tirtha appears to have been an even more direct source of inspiration. It seems probable that Yogananda's unexpected desire to join an agricultural education program in Japan before he made known his desire to travel to America may have been reinforced by Rama Tirtha's trajectory, which, like Vivekananda before him, took him through Japan into a two-year lecture tour across the United States. Satyananda recounts that Yogananda

> came to greatly appreciate the writings and teachings of the eminent Swami Rama Tirtha on Oneness, Non-Duality and Radiant Beingness. At that time, he always carried an English version of a condensed biography and/or book of sayings by Swami Rama Tirtha with him. The influence of that went to America with him.[22]

Yogananda was particularly fond of Rama Tirtha's poetry, much of which he translated into English and even set to music. The translations, in addition to more implicit influence, account for much of the material that is contained in his second publication, *Songs of the Soul* (1923).

Yogananda also cultivated some interesting connections with various exponents of universalist neo-Hinduism as well as more traditional notions of *sanātana dharma*. He used to be a regular visitor to the Nabo Bidhan Samāj in Calcutta, an offshoot organization of the original Brahmo Samāj founded by Keshub Chandra Sen, which emphasized a universal religion based on the synthesis of Hinduism—specifically yoga and Vaiṣṇava devotionalism—and Christian traditions. There he made the acquaintance of Jnananjan Niyogi, a political activist and social reformer who appears to have been the first to spark Yogananda's interest in education. Satyananda also claims that Niyogi's work would become helpful to Yogananda once he found himself in America, though the nature of this helpfulness is indeterminable and one can only assume that Satyananda is referring to some aspect of Niyogi's participation in the syncretic ideology of Sen's organization.

During this same time, Yogananda became exceedingly impressed by an encounter with a certain young Swami Dayananda.[23] Yogananda impulsively followed his new acquaintance to Benares in the company of another friend in 1909. Dayananda had made arrangements for both to be housed at the Bharat Dharma Mahamandal, though Yogananda quickly became disillusioned with the service-driven life of the ashram, which did not leave him much time for meditation. However, it was on this short-lived escape that Yogananda first encountered his future guru, Sri Yukteswar, who had actually been charged by Yogananda's concerned family with finding the would-be renunciant. Although Yogananda had been studying with Swami Kebalananda, another disciple of Lahiri Mahasaya also known as Shastri Mahasaya, he quickly decided that Sri Yukteswar was to be his true guru. Yogananda received initiation into the higher *kriyās* from Sri Yukteswar in that same year.

Becoming the International Yogi

Despite his voracious appetite for spiritual knowledge, Yogananda had a natural aversion to traditional education. At his family's urging, he enrolled at Sabour Agricultural College, which he quickly left, taking away only a large cabbage. He briefly entertained the idea of medical school, which never progressed beyond a stack of acquired and soon discarded reference materials. Finally, he enrolled at the Scottish Church College in Calcutta in 1910 at the insistence of both his family and Sri Yukteswar, who told him in no uncertain terms, "Someday you will go to the West. Its people will be more receptive to India's ancient wisdom if the strange Hindu teacher has a university degree."[24] It is unclear how much the "B.A.," which Yogananda dutifully appended to his name on the covers of his first several publications, really served to increase his credibility but he attained it nonetheless.

Yogananda's matriculation at the Scottish Church College did have one life-changing result. During his first year, he made the acquaintance of one Basu Kumar Bagchi, a man who under his future name of Swami Dhirananda would play an important if ultimately somewhat tragic role in Yogananda's life. Bagchi, who shared Yogananda's yogic interests, soon confided that he could not find a place at home that was private enough for proper meditation. Thenceforth, at Yogananda's insistence, Bagchi took up secret residence in his friend's attic meditation room. Eventually his presence inevitably became known to the Ghosh household, and he was duly integrated into the family.

Sri Yukteswar appears to have acknowledged from an early point in their relationship Yogananda's destiny—likely grounded in the latter's restless desire—to travel West. The teacher consequently attempted to groom his disciple to the best of his ability. He instructed Yogananda to read Vivekananda's works. Sri Yukteswar himself had been a fan of Vivekananda as well as Ramakrishna. He had once traveled to Dakshineswar to meet Ramakrishna, but for unspecified reasons the latter was not on site at the time and the meeting did not occur. Later, however, Sri Yukteswar would occasionally mingle with Ramakrishna's disciples, Swamis Vivekananda, Brahmananda, and Sivananda. He especially praised Vivekananda's spirit of nationalism. At one time, there was even a plan to integrate his organization as a department of the Ramakrishna Mission. Satyeswarananda recounts:

> He [Sri Yukteswar] had an idea that Sat Sanga Sova could become one department of the Sri Ramakrisna Mission, especially propagating yoga, since the Sri Ramakrisna Mission did not teach yoga. He met with Swami Brahmananda, the first president, to discuss the idea, but it did not materialize.[25]

Besides his concern to fill the Ramakrishna Mission's apparent lacuna, Sri Yukteswar's attempted merger was also motivated by a desire to prevent any future competition between Vivekananda's legacy and Yogananda. Sri Yukteswar "was aware that Yogananda might be envious of the image of Swami Vivekananda, because of Yogananda's ambition of wanting to be great,"[26] and he wished that his disciple might instead benefit from the other Yogi's teachings. The long shadow of Vivekananda would indeed become a particular point of inspiration for Yogananda, never quite amounting to outright rivalry but occasionally betraying a tinge of ambitious one-upmanship.

After transferring to the Serampore branch of the College of Calcutta in order to be closer to Sri Yukteswar's ashram, Yogananda finally received his degree in 1915 and entered the monastic order immediately thereafter. During this time, he had begun to express a restlessness with his native country. One imagines it was this same restlessness that caused him, in 1916, to enroll in an agricultural program in Japan that was aimed at educating young Bengalis abroad. With the exception of his brief and unproductive stint at the Sabour Agricultural College, Yogananda had never expressed any overwhelming passion for agriculture. In all likelihood, he had been hoping that Japan would serve as a launching pad to further adventures, just as it had for others in the past like Rama Tirtha and would again in the future for his own brother Bishnu Ghosh, as well as the latter's disciple, Bikram Choudhury.

Yogananda thus began preparations to travel abroad for the first time:

> Under the supervision of [his friend] Amar Mitra, Yogananda's new suit
> had been tailored. His hair was handsomely cut. Yogananda again became
> Mukundalal Ghosh . . . Guru Maharaj [Sri Yukteswar] had the desire that
> Yogananda at least keep his turban instead of donning a cap, but that was
> not possible.[27]

The whole affair, however, proved somewhat anticlimactic. Yogananda spent no
more than a week in Japan before boarding the next ship back to India. His close
friends had only just mailed off the first round of letters inquiring about his new
situation when he suddenly reappeared. According to Yogananda, he was immediately disenchanted by what he perceived as Japan's extremely "outward" lifestyle
and especially the "liberal mixing of men and women."[28] It is possible that the
four years that separated this trip from his later journey to the United States had
softened his standards, since it is unlikely that he would have found the American
lifestyle comparatively more conservative. It is perhaps more likely that he simply found himself disillusioned with the opportunities that Japanese agricultural
program could provide him in his yogic quest. His own *Autobiography* makes
no mention of the program and instead frames the sudden trip as a distressed
response to his oldest brother's failing health. Nevertheless, the trip was not
altogether a waste. On the returning ship to India, Yogananda encountered an
American couple who became quite fascinated with his expositions on monism
and the oneness of all religions and encouraged him to come to the United States.
These conversations would become the basis of Yogananda's first publication, *The
Science of Religion*, which he then and there resolved to write.

It would be another four years before Yogananda would follow the advice of
his American acquaintances. Upon his return to India, he busied himself with
the development of his school. The Yogoda Satsanga Brahmacharya Vidyalaya
was first founded in 1916, its initial location being in Calcutta at the home of
Tulsi Narayana Bose. Soon after, the establishment was moved to Dihika when
patronage was obtained from Maharaja Chandra Nandy of the Kasimbazar
Estate and then to Ranchi after a few of the students contracted malaria.[29] In
1920, however, news came of an International Conference of Religious Liberals in
Boston. Brahmo Samāj leader Herambra Chandra Maitra was to be the executive
member from India. At the time Maitra was also principal of the City College of
Calcutta, where Satyananda was one of his students. Satyananda requested that
Maitra submit Yogananda's name as the delegate from India, and it was subsequently arranged that Yogananda would travel to the conference to present on
the subject matter of *The Science of Religion* (1920), which was speedily completed

with the help of Bagchi (now Swami Dhirananda) and published with the aid of Satyananda and Bose. Soon thereafter, Yogananda set out from Calcutta to Boston on *The City of Sparta*, arriving to deliver his lecture on October 6, 1920.

Yogananda spent the first two years of his American residency in Boston. There, despite initially empty lecture halls, he managed to gather several key disciples who would be instrumental in the growth of his following and his later success. Alice Hasey, later initiated by Yogananda into Kriya Yoga as Yogamata, was particularly helpful in these early days, inviting Yogananda to live in her Boston home. On Christmas Eve 1920, Yogananda met Dr. Minott W. Lewis, a Boston dentist who, along with his wife Mildred, would become one of Yogananda's earliest and possibly closest American disciples. Mildred Lewis, who was a friend of Alice Hasey, was actually the first to see Yogananda when the two women attended one of his lectures at their local church. Yogananda would subsequently live in the Lewis household for nearly three years.

During this time, Yogananda appeared regularly at Unitarian Churches in the area and was eventually able to establish a small center overlooking Mystic Lake. Wendell Marshall Thomas, who included Yogananda in the 1930 book based on his doctoral dissertation, *Hinduism Invades America*, describes what must have been a fairly typical lecture that he himself attended. The event was held the Union Methodist Episcopal Church in New York City, cosponsored by the Dharma Mandal, or Fellowship of Faiths. The main floor of the church was "comfortably filled" with women and a "sprinkling" of men, some of whom were Hindus. There was an organ recital, an Episcopal rector offered a prayer for unity among men, and then a representative of the Dharma Mandal read a short play. After a call for participants in a staging of the aforementioned play and some advertisements of Yogananda's books and an English universalist journal, Yogananda was called up to speak:

> Yogananda was introduced as an Indian lecturer, writer and philosopher. As he rose from his seat in the audience to mount the platform, several persons in the audience rose also, perhaps out of gratitude for some benefit conferred by Yogoda, perhaps in honor of the spirituality of the East, perhaps in accord with the Indian pupil's respect for his master. The swami is short and plump, with a striking face. His raven hair hung over his shoulders in wavy locks—even longer than is usual among Bengalis—and he wore the vivid orange over his Western attire. His first act was to read one of his own poems, which he called "The Royal Sly Eluder," a record of his personal search for God in ocean, tree and sky, a search which ended in hearing God's voice within the soul, calling out "Hello, playmate, here am I!" The swami's voice was loud and clear, his pronunciation good. He then

began his demonstration of the "metaphysical unity of Hinduism and Christianity."

. . .

The preacher of the evening surely had his audience with him—at least its audible members. Clearly they felt in him a source of truth and comfort, inspiration and stimulation. They nodded assent to his pronouncements and laughed heartily at his jokes, especially when he called Christian preachers "spiritual victrolas" and proclaimed that Christianity was suffering from "theological indigestion."[30]

Although Thomas does not specify the year this lecture took place, based on the published books that kindled his interest in Yogananda it must have taken place sometime between 1926 and 1929,[31] likely during Yogananda's return to the East Coast after the opening of his Los Angeles center. This time frame would be reflective of a more established point in Yogananda's career (see fig. 3.1). His personal letters to Dr. Lewis make reference to earlier—and more difficult—days, when he would lecture to largely empty halls.[32]

Nevertheless, Yogananda's enterprise must have undergone significant growth even in its first two years, as evidenced by his letter to Satyananda:

Look. You all know that I can do the work of propagation, and people do come together, but running it in an orderly fashion is something I cannot write about. So, either Dhirananda or Satyananda, one of the two of you

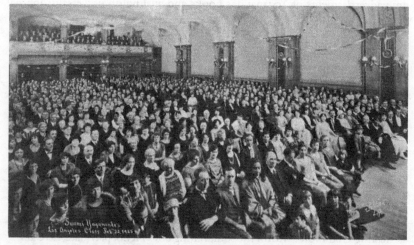

FIGURE 3.1 Yogananda's audience in Los Angeles on February 22, 1925, in *East-West* 1(1)

will have to come here to join in this work with huge potential. Both of you, be ready. Whomever I call will have to come without delay.[33]

Satyananda, being too busy with Sri Yukteswar's various projects as well as the management of Yogananda's Ranchi school, expressed his wish to remain in India, which was a disappointment to Yogananda. Dhirananda set off to the United States in 1922 in his stead and for the next seven years would be indispensable in promoting and maintaining Yogananda's organization and helping with his numerous lectures and publications.

Yogananda began to expand his lecture campaign in late 1923 and early 1924, traveling to give multiple lectures in New York. There he met Mohammed Rashid, who at the time had just completed his university degree but had in fact arrived in America four years earlier on the very same ship that carried Yogananda there. Rashid, who had been intrigued by Yogananda's teachings even when he had briefly encountered the Swami on board the boat, became a kind of secretary to him. In this capacity Rashid took on the promotional aspects of Yogananda's campaign. Reportedly, he was in fact responsible for the majority of Yogananda's rather sensational posters during this period, which Yogananda in fact objected to as he considered them to be "fulsome."[34]

The publicity did prove to be effective, despite Yogananda's misgivings, and he quickly became a well-known lecturer and a favorite of New York high society. No doubt Rashid, who appeared to be endowed with a certain acumen for representation, was instrumental in Yogananda's already ongoing adaptation to the American social climate. According to Satyeswarananda, "When Yogananda realized after Capt. Rashid had joined him that a poor looking man could not expect social recognition in that affluent country, he gradually turned himself into an affluent person."[35] Although Satyeswarananda is arguably the most critical biographer in his accounts of Yogananda—especially with respect to his Westernization of Kriya Yoga practice and fondness for organizations—there must have been some truth to this observation. As actress Shirley MacLaine would inform Bikram Choudhury some half-a-century later, "in America, if you don't charge money . . . people won't respect you."[36] Yogananda waged something of a personal war with materialism for the rest of his life—acquiring what was, according to the *Los Angeles Times*, a "swanky automobile" but giving away his stylish new overcoat. The affluent air of his Mt. Washington and Encinitas estates, even as he was still receiving aid from his father in India and scraping together funds from his wealthy disciples, illustrates that he came to fully internalize the idea that in America even spiritual capital was difficult to accrue without the backing of material wealth.

Rashid, true to his enthusiasm for promotion, soon encouraged Yogananda to expand his campaign even further, pushing him to deliver his lectures across the United States. A car was purchased and in 1924—accompanied by Rashid, disciple Arthur Cometer, and another driver only known as Ralph—Yogananda set out on a cross-continental lecture tour. Having traveled across the country, Yogananda sailed to Alaska before returning to lecture in Seattle and Portland, and proceeding down the California coast to Los Angeles. It was here that his sights settled on a particularly attractive house at the top of Mt. Washington.

Yogananda developed a great fondness for Los Angeles, to which he famously liked to refer as the "Benares of America," and more generally claimed that "you can practice yoga better in California than anywhere else on earth. The climate is more conducive."[37] The purchasing of the house on Mt. Washington was funded by several separate contributions, some of which seemed to have magically materialized at the very last imaginable moment. After a bit of financial and legal wrangling, Yogananda established the headquarters of his Yogoda Satsanga at the Mt. Washington estate, which was officially inaugurated on October 25, 1925. After a brief sojourn at the newly established center, Yogananda departed on another promotional lecture tour. Dhirananda, who had by this time comfortably established himself in the intellectual circles of Boston, was called upon to drop everything to take up management of the establishment.

The "Ire of 200 Husbands" and the "Swami Row"

The first of the above headlines appeared on February 4, 1928, discretely tucked away on page thirteen of the Los Angeles Times. In Florida, however, Yogananda was making front-page news. In keeping with a persistent American nervousness regarding the Yogi's sexuality, Yogananda faced no shortage of accusations regarding the nature of his teachings. One particularly illustrative—and well-documented—incident occurred upon one of his returns to the East Coast following the establishment of the Mt. Washington center. Yogananda had been scheduled to deliver a series of lectures in Miami. However, the first lecture appears to have had an impact sensational enough to render any further arrangements rather impossible.

Following a number of complaints, Yogananda was accused by the Miami police of accepting thirty-five dollars each from some 200 women for private lessons in the secrets of his "mystic cult." The newspapers overflowed with stories of domestic conflict wrought by unruly wives insistent on attending Yogananda's lectures. A distressed son found his mother, who was subsequently hospitalized, trying to walk on the Miami River because "Yogananda told her she could do it."[38] Impoverished women were allegedly borrowing thirty-five dollars just to attend the Swami's lecture. Yogananda, for his part, denied that he had given any private lessons in Miami, said that the woman who had been hospitalized had been suffering for twenty years and came to him with the consent of her husband, and specified that, besides, he charged only twenty-five dollars for his lectures. Yogananda was nevertheless blocked by the police department from delivering any subsequent presentations. The Miami police chief, Leslie Quigg, claimed that his prohibiting Yogananda from holding any further events was due to no personal grudge against the Swami but rather in the interest of public order and Yogananda's own safety. Quigg reportedly had received multiple phone calls containing veiled threats against Yogananda and promising that if the police did not ensure that the "cult leader" left town, others would take matters into their own hands.

Unwilling to concede defeat, Yogananda attempted to obtain a restraining order that would stop the police from further interfering with his scheduled lectures. It was then explicitly "suggested" that Yogananda leave Miami. The lecture hall was surrounded by police armed with tear gas to prevent any person from entering, whether to deliver a lecture or to observe one. Police Chief Quigg expressed concerns about riots. After a lengthy and sensationalized appeals process, Yogananda was nevertheless unable to deliver his lectures as planned. As the news reports of these proceedings suggest, Yogananda appeared to have left quite an impression on Miami's female population.

The reports especially honed in on the unfortunate progress of one woman— name not provided—who had apparently experienced a total mental break and been confined to a sanitarium following Yogananda's lecture, described by her family physician as "violently insane." Sanitarium director Charles A. Reed further testified:

> She talks about the Swami constantly and imagines she is a lion, attempting to roar and conduct herself as she thinks a lion does. . . . She says the Swami told her he was a lion and that he had Miami in his grasp. She refuses food until attendants assure her it has been in contact with the Swami and she insists it must be of the proper color and proper vibrations.[39]

The woman's husband testified that although she had previously been a Spiritualist and trance medium, she had been mentally and physically sound until she attended Yogananda's lectures. Numerous witnesses testified in defense of Yogananda, claiming that his lectures had in fact been highly spiritual in character and had contained no objectionable elements. A Presbyterian minister who had come all the way from Philadelphia even declared that Yogananda's explanations of the sayings of Jesus were the purest and best he had ever heard. However, on cross-examination he was forced to admit that Yogananda had not based his lectures on texts from the Bible although he did make frequent use of quotations from it.

A local pastor, Revered R. N. Merrill, then testified that he had been called upon to counsel a woman whose relatives insisted she was under Yogananda's hypnotic spell. In a similar spirit, it was speculated that Yogananda had attempted to hypnotize Police Chief Quigg as well. One report states that "seated across the table at the police station, the Hindu philosopher gazed dreamily into the eyes of Chief Quigg in an effort to mesmerize him, but the hypnotic influences were sharply interrupted when the chief ordered him to stop."[40] In response to these accusations, in his final rebuttal, Yogananda insisted that he condemned hypnotism, explaining that he practiced magnetism, which was an "entirely different thing." Without attributing any truth to these accusations one way or another, one is nevertheless tempted to wonder at the correspondence between these accusations as being par for the course amidst a bout of sensationalized Yogi phobia and Yogananda's actual experimentations with hypnotism in his youth. It would appear that at least at one time he too thought that such practices were well within the purview of what it meant to be a Yogi.

Even more incendiary than the possibility of hypnotism was the overwhelmingly female constitution of Yogananda's audience. Yogananda's organization was repeatedly referred to as a "love cult" and presented as part of a sort of rising epidemic, as evidenced by the fact that just a few months prior to the Miami incident, authorities in Switzerland had "uncovered sensational activities of an allegedly similar organization in the Alps, where east Indian teachers and their feminine followers disported themselves in the nude."[41] If such implicit connections were not damning enough, the papers further cited accusations that Yogananda had already been chased out of Los Angeles after having his nose broken by an insulted husband.

Although Yogananda firmly refuted this alleged altercation as a slanderous case of mistaken identity, his connection to the incident was closer than his denials implied. The man for whom Yogananda had been mistaken was none other than Dhirananda, who during Yogananda's absence had been placed in charge of the Mt. Washington center and was therefore forced to shoulder the responsibility when its activities came under scrutiny. Indeed, some three weeks before Yogananda's own unfortunate brush with an angry mob in Miami, Dhirananda had to be escorted off a train when he returned from the East Coast to Los Angeles so as to keep reporters at bay in light of the District Attorney's investigation of the center.

Contrary to Yogananda's claims that he had been in no way implicated in the Los Angeles scandal, his own role in the matter was under just as much scrutiny as Dhirananda's. If Dhirananda was the presiding chief of an organization where "a love-cult [was] being conducted under the cloak of the Vedantic religion of India," then Yogananda was similarly guilty as the "writer of various books and pamphlets in which an unusual philosophy of love and sex control are declared to be unfolded."[42] Yogananda wisely chose to remain in Washington, DC, at that time. Unsurprisingly, the District Attorney's concern was specifically over whether young women had been present at the various classes during which "theories" of love and sex had been discussed. It is not possible to determine whether the center had ever actually offered any such classes, though it seems doubtful given the general tone of Yogananda's teachings and especially the conservative attitude of Dhirananda.

Nevertheless, as in the case of his early experimentation with hypnotism, there is some evidence to suggest that Yogananda did not altogether renounce the persona of the lascivious Yogi. Only a year after the "love-cult" scandals, Dhirananda left Yogananda and the Mt. Washington center. He lectured under his own name in the Los Angeles area. His advertisements often appeared only inches from Yogananda's in the papers, and the *Los Angeles Times* profiled him as one of the city's most influential Swamis alongside Yogananda and Paramananda in 1932. In December 1932, Dhirananda abandoned his Swami title altogether and entered the University of Iowa to pursue a doctorate in electroencephalography. A subsequent 1935 lawsuit by Dhirananda—now once more Basu Kumar Bagchi—would raise questions as to whether his departure was in some way prompted by sexual indiscretions on Yogananda's part. The lawsuit dealt more specifically with a promissory note that Dhirananda had "coerced" Yogananda to sign as a form of remuneration and severance when Dhirananda unexpectedly appeared at Yogananda's New York apartment before returning to Los Angeles and officially leaving the organization.

The newspapers scrambled to cover the sensational "Swami Row,"[43] which was presented as a squabble over money and a bruised ego. Dhirananda cited his and Yogananda's mutual cooperation at the Ranchi school and his subsequent journey to America at Yogananda's request, which he consented to only after Yogananda had imploringly sent him the passage money. However, Dhirananda claimed that ultimately he "found a disgusting situation. . . . He [Yogananda] had given people the impression that I was as a foundling, a puny little boy that he might have found in the gutter. He was my preceptor here, although in India I held higher scholastic degrees and received higher salaries."[44] Yet it had taken Dhirananda a full seven years of dutiful cooperation to become unsatisfied with this state of affairs, which raises the question of whether the "disgusting situation" that had spurred him to action was something other than a lack of proper recognition from his associate.

The court proceedings indicate that Yogananda filed a counter-suit when Dhirananda finally attempted to collect the amount of the promissory note after finishing his degree in 1935. Yogananda's counter-suit claimed that the note was wrongfully extorted under threat of defaming his name and reputation by releasing fabricated information to the press and additionally falsely charging that Dhirananda was his associate and partner in the publication of *The Science of Religion* as well as the *Yogoda* pamphlets.[45] The latter set of "false" charges is actually historically true—Dhirananda was credited on the covers of both publications as Yogananda's "Associate." It would not be unreasonable to imagine that Dhirananda's threats of defamation may have also had some roots in actual events or, at least, Dhirananda's belief that such events had occurred. Rumors have since circulated in the SRF community that Dhirananda's unexpected visit to New York was prompted by hints that he might discover Yogananda's living situation to be highly problematic. Other rumors have claimed that Dhirananda actually arrived to discover Yogananda sharing his apartment with a woman. No official claims concerning such matters were ever made by Dhirananda himself. Yogananda spent the duration of the lawsuit in India and later in Mexico. Directly prior to leaving the country in 1935, Yogananda incorporated the Self-Realization Fellowship as a nonprofit organization and reassigned all of his property, including Mt. Washington, to the corporation, thereby protecting his assets.

Such accusations would resurface with greater specificity when Nirad Ranjan Chowdhury, Yogananda's new associate, left in a strikingly similar manner ten years later. Chowdhury was brought in to take over Dhirananda's role in directing the center only months after the latter's departure. Under the name Sri Nerode, he taught at and maintained the Mt. Washington center and also toured the lecture-circuit with Yogananda and his associates for the next decade. Chowdhury had attended the University of Calcutta and subsequently traveled to the United States to study Sanskrit at Harvard and Berkeley. He first encountered Yogananda at public lectures in Boston and San Francisco in the early 1920s and subsequently became head of a newly established Yogoda center in Detroit in 1926. Chowdhury never took any formal vows and was thus known as Sri Nerode (an Anglicization of his first name) or Brahmachari Nerode. By 1929, when Yogananda called upon him to take the reins at Mt. Washington, Chowdhury was heading Yogoda centers at Detroit and Pittsburgh, had published two small books advertised in Yogananda's *East-West* magazine, and was lecturing extensively both at the centers and other locations across the country. In 1932 Chowdhury, who was now married and recently a father, set off on a promotional tour that lasted until 1937, when the family returned to Mt. Washington.

All appeared to be well until in October 1939 the newspapers exploded with stories of a half-million-dollar lawsuit filed by Chowdhury against Yogananda. Like Dhirananda before him, Chowdhury left the SRF, leveling a number of accusations against his former friend and colleague. There is some speculation that the accusations, which were quite inflammatory, were never meant to be publicized but rather were intended to serve as a warning to Yogananda and were only leaked to the press due to a mistake made by Chowdhury's lawyer. In any case, according to the *Los Angeles Times*, Chowdhury charged that Yogananda "preferred the company of young women students to the practice of his religious offices" and had "taken to holding himself up before his students as a sort of deity and has advocated that they live on below-normal rations of food and submit to other self-denials while he himself 'hypocritically' lived a life of luxury." Even more damning were reports that young female disciples were placed closer to Yogananda's quarters at Mt. Washington while older women lived in more distant spaces, and Yogananda himself "occupie[d] an apartment house wherein girls are seen dashing in and out at all times of the day and night."[46] Chowdhury sued for $500,000 in damages, alleging that Yogananda had told him that he considered him a partner in the SRF—which Yogananda had offhandedly valued at one million dollars—after Chowdhury had saved Mt. Washington from certain financial collapse.[47] One suspects that the sum was chiefly symbolic.

In later coverage of the trial, presumably once the initial flood of sensational allegations was suppressed, Chowdhury's claims became limited to accusing Yogananda of "teaching doctrines diametrically opposed to those of the Hindu self-realization philosophy" and "conducting his life in a manner 'repugnant' to the interests and objects of the partnership," adding that "the swami ha[d] attempted to gain control over his—Chowdhury's—personal affairs and those of his family in a manner which has destroyed the partnership's harmony."[48] In any case, the suit was dismissed when Yogananda produced a written statement made by Chowdhury in 1929 stating that he would be offering his labors to the SRF *pro bono*. Presumably Yogananda had learned something from his earlier legal wrangling with Dhirananda.

Yogananda himself had consistently cautioned his disciples against unruly sexuality. Kriyananda writes that the Swami would sometimes quote the following statement, once told to him by a saint:

Woman leads a twofold existence. During the day, she is sweet and pleasing to look at. Thus, she lures men into her trap. At night, however, she becomes a tigress and drinks man's blood!

Did you know that one seminal emission is equal to losing a quart of blood? It saps your power. There *is* power in that fluid; there has to be. It was given you to create new life.[49]

Whether or not Yogananda himself had ever created new life remains a deep controversy. In 1995 a son of one of Yogananda's devotees brought a lawsuit claiming that Yogananda was his biological father. The suit was settled in 2002 when DNA evidence submitted by the SRF showed no biological relationship. The validity of this same DNA evidence is hotly contested within the community of Yogananda's detractors.

The Man with Superpowers

When it comes to the matter of superpowers, Yogananda's *Autobiography* tells a double-layered narrative. Although the earlier chapters are full of spectacular feats performed by Yogis making cameo-style appearances and accounts of power displayed by Yogananda's guru Sri Yukteswar and his guru Lahiri Mahasaya, Yogananda generally diminishes the significance of powers in the later parts of his book, focusing instead on metaphysics and the evolution of his spiritual understanding. There are no more superpowers on American soil. In proper fashion, he certainly claims none for himself. Yet the historical evidence suggests that Yogananda's youthful fascination with superpowers—including cultivating some of his own—followed him well into adulthood and his American career.

To his followers, Yogananda was a man of paradox. His casual student Hilda Charlton describes a fedora-wearing Yogananda whose eyes would light up with delight over the novelty of a garbage disposal[50] even as she acknowledges his evident mental powers. Kriyananda—who, like Davis, met Yogananda in 1948 after reading his *Autobiography*—talks of Yogananda as a kind-hearted trickster who in his childhood caused the family cook's hand to stick to a wall after the man had teased him about his meditation practice. He also attributes to Yogananda such feats as healing with the touch of his hand, levitating during meditation, pacifying a tiger with a mere glance, and smuggling Mexican mangoes into California using a Jedi-style mind trick. With the exception of the mango incident, however, these are not occurrences that Kriyananda himself witnessed, though he does recount a number of "miracles" performed by Yogananda in his presence, which generally tend to fall into the realm of synchronicity. Kriyananda attributes these abilities to "magnetism,"[51] a term which Yogananda himself used and, as discussed earlier, was quite careful to distinguish from hypnotism and Mesmerism. Kriyananda is careful to avoid stating that magnetism has any direct influence on the psychologies of others but rather explains it as a method of "attracting," by the sheer force of one's will, desired effects.

Dr. Lewis captures both the playfulness of Yogananda's character and his aura of power when he describes their relationship as follows:

> As I have said, many nights were spent in listening to his wonderful words and his experiences and romping about the house as brothers keeping

Mrs. Lewis in a state of turmoil—which seemed to be just what we wanted; but in spite of all those things, that wonderful reverence and devotion was never tainted in the least bit; and the Master was our Master in spite of the close relationship.[52]

Lewis attributes great charisma and spiritual gravitas to Yogananda. Where he addresses specific superhuman abilities that his teacher has exhibited, they generally have to do with healing.

Yogananda was also known to engage in some markedly more ostentatious displays of power, at times blurring the line between demonstrations of mental control or magnetism and stage magic. Charlton describes a lecture that Yogananda delivered in Oakland, where his talk focused on the importance of bodily control:

He interrupted his talk to ask if there was a doctor in the audience. A man stood up and Swamiji asked him to come on the stage. He requested the doctor, "Take my pulse and tell me what you feel." The doctor felt his wrist, looking perplexed at first and then amazed. "There is no pulse," he answered. Swamiji then told him to take the pulse on the other wrist. The doctor's facial expression turned from amazement to incredulity. He said, "Swami Yogananda, this is impossible. Your pulse is pounding at an incredible speed." He quickly tried the other side again and said, "This side is normal." He came down from the stage into the audience shaking his head and mumbling, "Impossible, impossible."[53]

Later on in the same lecture Yogananda sent six men catapulting across the stage with a mere straightening of his body and a flick of his stomach.[54] Without making any claims concerning the authenticity of Yogananda's superpowers, it should be noted that the first phenomenon involving his pulse is consistent with a very common stage trick performed by placing a ball, lemon, or other small spherical object under the armpit so as to cut off the circulation to one arm. The latter demonstration has a similar performative history, though it tends less towards stage magic and more toward iron-man acts. Other demonstrations drew even more explicitly on physical culture and especially on the more visually impressive elements of *haṭha* yogic *āsana* practice. As early as 1923, after demonstrating a version of the stomach-flicking act using a large sofa, Yogananda "squatted on the floor, and in an instant had his toes curled up in his lap. . . . To show how far such techniques may be carried, Yogananda proceeded to curl himself into a ball, and raise his body on his two hands."[55] While Yogananda's lectures were not generally advertised as exhibitions of superhuman power, it is not uncommon to see promises of "Prayer Vibrations" and "Divine Healing by Holy Ghost Christ Power and Yogi Method" among the listed attractions (fig. 3.2).

Yogananda's lecture announcements frequently represented him as imparting the secrets of "Miracle-Working Yogis of a Land of Mystery," occasionally declaring that these would be accompanied by "Amazing Demonstrations of Recharging the Body Batteries." While the actual "recharging" may have been effected by a combination of meditation and *prāṇāyāma*, these techniques do not make for a very convincing demonstration. On the other hand, it seems that sending six men flying across a stage would adequately prove that one's body batteries were, so to speak, fully charged.

Outside of his own performances, it appears that Yogananda would occasionally bring in external talent in the form of a colorful cast of collaborators. The most long-lived of these associations was with Yogi Hamid Bey, who later, sans his Yogi title, went on to found the Coptic Fellowship. His biography, as propagated by the organization, claims that Bey hailed from Egypt, where he spent his childhood and early youth studying with a master at a Coptic Christian temple. After

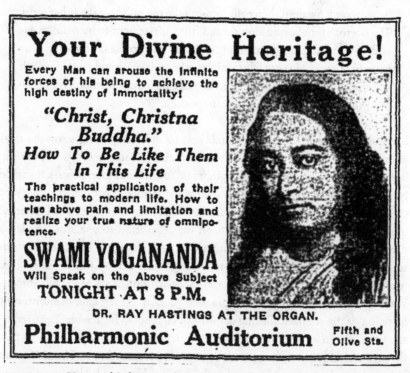

FIGURE 3.2 Yogananda's lecture advertisement in the *Los Angeles Times*, October 13, 1925

serving in the armed forces during World War I, he traveled to Italy to demonstrate his powers to the world in order to reveal the true nature of human ability.

His performances attracted the attention of famous stage-magician Harry Houdini, who claimed that he could replicate Bey's state of suspended animation, which had purportedly allowed him to survive a three-hour burial, through the use of shallow breathing. Bey was invited to the United States in 1926 to face off against Houdini, but the latter died a mere three weeks after Bey arrived. However, in January 1927 Bey nevertheless performed his demonstration in the presence of the media, several doctors, and a small crowd in northern New Jersey, officially beating Houdini's record. Bey emerged from his grave three hours after being interred, his ears, nose, and mouth still stuffed with cotton, the sand placed on his face undisturbed, and his pulse as steady as when he had entered the grave.[56] Following this performance, Bey toured the vaudeville circuit for a number of years, during which time he appears to have made the acquaintance of Yogananda.

Yogananda encountered Bey in Buffalo in mid-1927. He describes his new associate, the "Miracle Man," as follows:

I was quite impressed with the beautiful spiritual gleam in Mr. Bey's eyes. I sang the song, "O God Beautiful!" for him. Ever since then he has been singing it. Hamid Bey is an Egyptian from the Soudan, famous land of sheiks. He was reared under an austere mystical training, and the feats he performs are a part of the religious rites of his sect. Mr. Bey showed me that by touching anyone's wrist he could divine his thoughts.

. . .

Later, he demonstrated to me his method of physical trance, in which he fell into my hands, breathless and almost lifeless. The stethoscope revealed that his heart-beat, at first fast, slowed down to an intermittent beat, and then got very slow. Mr. Bey can remain underground, buried for twenty-four hours, sealed in an air-tight casket, and can hold a thousand pounds on his chest. He controls his pulse at will—its beats appeared and completely disappeared at his will. He also pierces his body with long needles without bloodshed. The marks almost instantaneously disappeared after the needles were withdrawn. He thrusts these needles into his throat, cheeks and tongue without pain. He can produce blood from one puncture and withhold blood from another. Most of these things he performed right in front of me. In the various cities where he visits he often gives demonstrations before gatherings of eminent physicians and surgeons.

. . .

Passing needles thru his cheeks and certain other of Mr. Bey's feats are performed, after long practice, by manipulating glands of the throat and

by pressing certain nerves on the head. These are very interesting physiological phenomena showing that man can control the functions of the
heart and all other organs of involuntary action. This is known to Hindu
Yogis and Swamis who practice Yoga, as well as to mystics of other sects.
Of course, it must be remembered that without the love of God and without wisdom, such control and feats are just physiological jugglery and a
detriment to spiritual realization. . . . I told Mr. Bey to produce trance
by love of God, rather than merely by glandular pressure, as results produced by devotion are safer and greater. Generally, it takes another person
to arouse Mr. Bey from his trance. But, in the conscious trance of devotion, or Yoga, one never loses consciousness but transcends the material
consciousness and comes back to consciousness of matter at will again.
That is the conscious communion with God the Yogoda aspires to teach.[57]

It is unclear whether Bey ever managed to induce the trance state with no
aid from glandular manipulation, but Yogananda appears to have been satisfied enough with his progress to incorporate the performance into his lectures.
Bey delivered a number of presentations alongside Yogananda including some
of the very same burial demonstrations—though significantly truncated for the
sake of the audience's patience. Chowdhury, who was at this time still affiliated
with Yogananda, also lectured together with Bey. Bey was made an Honorary
Vice-President of the SRF in 1933 and maintained some form of affiliation with
Yogananda until he returned to Egypt in 1936 and thereafter set off to found his
own organization in 1937 (figs. 3.3 and 3.4).

Another associate of Yogananda's was Roman Ostoja. Ostoja first emerged
as a contact of Yogananda in 1934, when the two collaborated on at least one
series of lectures in Oakland. Billed as Yogi R. Ostoja for the purposes of these
presentations, he elsewhere went by Notredameus and represented himself as
a Polish count, though this claim to nobility is unsubstantiated. That he was at
least of Polish descent is almost certain. Sources indicate that he immigrated to
the United States from Poland in 1923 as Mieszko Roman Maszerski and subsequently petitioned for naturalization in Southern California in 1934, around
the time that he would have made Yogananda's acquaintance. As early as 1931,
however, Ostoja had been making a name for himself in the Los Angeles area as
a medium, a hypnotist—though he appears to have worked mostly with domestic animals and birds—and a performer of typical attractions such as suspended
animation, lying on a bed of nails, and piercing his tongue and hands with metal
spikes. There he also befriended the famous author Upton Sinclair, who at the
time was exploring telepathy and Spiritualism, and he even attempted to perform
a séance that included Albert Einstein as part of the audience.

BEGINNING TONIGHT !!!

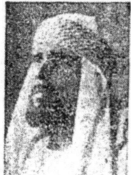

YOGI HAMID BEY

Have you found your true vocation in life? Do you know how to blow away your troubles? Can you rejuvenate yourself at will? Do you know how to have greatest happiness with your family? Do you know how to know your true mate in marriage? Can you overcome susceptibility to diseases?

Learn Complete Control of your Body, Mind and Soul from a Master Yogi,

HAMID BEY

WHO CAN DEMONSTRATE WHAT HE TEACHES

The only Yogi to be introduced by

SWAMI YOGANANDA

WHO SPEAKS ON

"What Happens 10 Minutes After Death."

SEE YOGI BURY HIMSELF ALIVE TONIGHT

WEDNESDAY, April 8th, 8 P.M.

Demonstrations and Lectures on April 8, 9, 10, 11 and 12.

TRINITY AUDITORIUM

Office: 227 Homer Laughlin Bldg., 315 South Broadway. MU. 5062.

FIGURE 3.3 Hamid Bey advertisement in the *Los Angeles Times*, April 8, 1931

TWO MORE NIGHTS

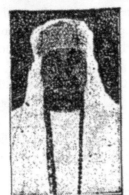

THE EXPERIENCE OF A LIFETIME

YOGI HAMID BEY

Miracle Man and Magnetic Healer from Egypt

Buries Himself Alive and Comes Back Alive

The Only Yogi to be Introduced by

SWAMI YOGANANDA

SATURDAY, APRIL 11TH, 8 P.M. Unusual demonstration of healing magnetism and science baffling demonstration of control of circulation by YOGI HAMID BEY.

SUNDAY, APRIL 12TH, 8 P.M. Demonstration of Science-baffling Telepathy and Conscious Burial by YOGI HAMID BEY who repeats all previous demonstrations this night.
Lecture on "MIRACLES OF SUPER-CONCENTRATION" by SWAMI YOGANANDA.

No matter what your diseases are, you will find help through these demonstrations and lectures. They will reveal surer methods of success.

TRINITY AUDITORIUM (9th and Grand)

FIGURE 3.4 Hamid Bey advertisement in the *Los Angeles Times*, April 11, 1931

Judging by his list of "stage" talents, Ostoja was something of a second Bey. Indeed, the lectures given by Yogananda alongside Ostoja's demonstrations were virtually identical to those presented with the support of Bey—the most memorable of these being titled "What Happens Ten Minutes After Death," which presumably played off of Bey's and Ostoja's common talent for being buried alive. The following announcement appeared in the *Berkeley Daily Gazette* on October 20, 1934:

> Dr. Roman Ostoja, sponsored by Swami Yogananda, founder of the Self Realization Fellowship of Los Angeles, will give a series of phenomenal self-mastery demonstrations and lectures at Ebell Hall, 1440 Harrison Street, Oakland, at 8 o'clock Sunday, Monday, and Wednesday evenings.
>
> His subjects will be:
>
> Sunday, "Science of Instantaneous Healing and Overcoming Nervousness," also Special Demonstrations.
>
> Monday, "What Happens Ten Minutes After Death."
>
> Wednesday, "Developing Magnetic Power of Will."
>
> Dr. Roman Ostoja is a Westerner. After undergoing rigorous training in the caves of wisdom in the Himalayas, his earnestness and sincerity were recognized by the masters of the Far East, and he was entrusted by them with the sacred mission of bringing the Divine teachings of the East to the Western people. He spent many years in working out a simplified method of instruction, a method which is adaptable to the westerner, yet does not destroy the essence of the eastern teachings.
>
> Since coming to this country, Dr. Roman Ostoja has appeared with his teachings and demonstrations before Harvard University, Columbia University, and Ann Harbor [*sic*], also University of Southern California, Los Angeles. He has also appeared before various medical and scientific groups and individuals, among them Albert Einstein. Everywhere he has received acknowledgement.
>
> He is not only lecturing and teaching, but demonstrating mental telepathy and death-defying feats which display so-called super-human powers. He performs these mental miracles to prove that a westerner is capable of controlling the infinite forces.

There is more no credible evidence as to whether Ostoja had studied with the Himalayan masters than that he was a Polish aristocrat, though the former seems even less likely than the latter, since it only becomes a prominent feature of Ostoja's advertised biography subsequent to his association with Yogananda.[58]

At this point, Ostoja's life story begins to mimic a Blavatskian trajectory—an already exotic Slavic nobleman, steeped in the wisdom of the Orient and charged with bringing the message to the Western masses. Particularly interesting is Ostoja's appropriation of the Yogi title, its use rationalized in the above announcement as demonstrating the transferability and therefore universality of yogic power. This was, of course, perfectly in tune with Yogananda's message, which sought to render the practice of yoga and the figure of the Yogi less foreign and to show that his potential was equally accessible to the Western disciple. At the time of his 1934 lectures, Ostoja was announced as the new head of the SRF's healing department. In subsequent years, Ostoja maintained some further affiliation with Yogananda, being listed as an ordained SRF minister in 1937. During this time, he also founded the short-lived Infinite Science Institute through which he propagated his own teachings.

Thus, in addition to occasional demonstrations of his own apparently superhuman abilities, Yogananda made an effort to surround himself with other exemplars of superpowerful human potential, who inevitably became billed as Yogis even if they had had no prior association with the title. Like Yogananda's own demonstrations, however, their displays were brought into alignment with his fundamental message that the Yogi's abilities are not only scientific but ultimately stem from a divine universal source. Bey's esoteric mastery of glands and nerves—which few of Yogananda's SRF disciples could hope to achieve—was subordinated in efficacy to love of God, which was stated to produce a superior version of the same effect. Ostoja's penchant for hypnotizing rabbits was swept under the rug, and he became instead the Western Yogi who healed thousands at every lecture. In what was perhaps a business-savvy fashion, Yogananda continuously sought to portray the Yogi's powers as formidable but not sinister, wondrous but not inaccessible.

Yogis Incorporated and a Return to the Land of Miracles

If there is one matter that alienates Yogananda—and therefore the SRF as well as its India-based branch, the Yogoda Satsanga Society (YSS)—from the other instantiations of the Kriya Yoga monastic lineage that traces itself through Lahiri Mahasaya's revelation from Babaji, it is the organized, almost corporate nature of Yogananda's legacy. Indeed, Yogananda's Indian biographers rarely miss an opportunity to pad their treatment of Yogananda's life's work with at least a light anti-organizational polemic. Satyananda's and especially Satyeswarananda's writings dwell much more extensively than Yogananda's *Autobiography* on the effort expended by Lahiri Mahasaya to convince Babaji to allow householders to be initiated into Kriya Yoga.

In alignment with this, Lahiri Mahasaya is characterized as being firmly against any organizations established for the purpose of propagating the tradition. Although he finally received Babaji's blessing to spread Kriya outside the strictly delimited ranks of initiated renunciants, he continued to emphasize the traditional mode of initiation and transmission centered on the personal relationship between guru and disciple. In 1885 the Arya Mission Institution was established with the permission of Lahiri Mahasaya by his chief disciple, Panchanan Bhattacharya. It was, however, made expressly clear that the purpose of the organization would be solely for the distribution of books about the general premises of Kriya and certain herbal medicines, but no actual instruction in Kriya practice would take place through the institution.

Sri Yukteswar was technically the first to break with this anti-institutionalism. He established two ashrams, which were partially used to propagate the teachings of Kriya but did not grant initiation independent of actual discipleship to Sri Yukteswar himself. As previously stated, Sri Yukteswar also at one time envisioned joining forces with the Ramakrishna Mission in order to offer instruction in yogic practice. This effort to stem a developing rivalry between Vivekananda's organization and his own disciple's ambitions was not unfounded. Satyeswarananda describes a young Yogananda who, standing on the bank of the Ganges at Dakshineswar across from the headquarters of the International Ramakrishna Mission and Math, firmly declared: "I will make mine bigger than theirs."[59]

Yogananda's ambitions began to reach fruition with the opening of the Mt. Washington Center in Los Angeles in 1925, under the name Yogoda Satsanga, which had already been used to designate Yogananda's school in Ranchi. Yogananda's *East-West*, later renamed *Self-Realization Fellowship Magazine*, made its debut this same year. To round matters out, around this same time Yogananda created his signature correspondence course. The course, which is still available by mail-order from the SRF, consists of a series of lessons ranging from health and diet to "talks on the development of the mind and heart, and visionary teachings on spiritual sadhana and other such things."[60] This idea was not entirely novel. Ramacharaka had also offered correspondence courses, and in 1910 the New Thought journal *Nautilus* advertised a yoga correspondence course by Sakharam Ganesh Pandit of Bombay, mailed every Thursday.[61] Nevertheless, the course was instrumental in spreading Yogananda's message and was indisputably representative of Yogananda's overall business model in approaching the dissemination of his message. Over the next decade, Yogoda centers were established in seventeen major cities throughout the United States as well as in several international locations. Yogananda listed three centers in India, including the Ranchi school, a Calcutta address, and Sri Yukteswar's Karar Ashram in Puri.

Incorporating his organization as the Self-Realization Fellowship in 1935 seems to have further fanned the flames of Yogananda's institutionalizing fervor. Upon returning to India later that year and seeing that Sri Yukteswar had been using the name "Yogad Satsanga" to advertise an aspect of his establishment, Yogananda excitedly announced his own desire to start an international organization called Yogoda Satsanga. This appeared to be a point of disagreement between him and Sri Yukteswar, who allegedly told his student: "You have your organization in the West, and I am going to nominate you as the next president of Sadhu Sova. So what more organizations do you need?"[62] It was also argued that the name—aside from being bad Sanskrit—would imply that Yogananda alone had started the organization, despite the presence of Satyananda and others. After some more debate, Sri Yukteswar finally agreed on the condition that Yogananda would list him as founder and himself as the first president, but, much to Sri Yukteswar's displeasure, Yogananda turned down this offer. Nevertheless, it appears that an agreement was ultimately reached and Sri Yukteswar's Yogad Sat Sanga Sova became the Yogoda Satsanga Society of India in 1936, which persists as the Indian branch of the SRF to this day. This latter point evidently created some bad blood between the Indian members of the Kriya lineage and the Western SRF management, and accounts of the institution's history abound with detailed cataloguing of changes in leadership and legal wrangles.

Yogananda made only one return visit to India during the three decades between his initial departure in 1920 and his death in 1952. While his 1935 homecoming was accompanied by grand fanfare, tensions simmered below the surface. Satyeswarananda recounts that "Yogananda's return to India somehow got bad press. Some people said: 'Swami is in big business in America.' Some of these people had connection with a group of people from Miami, in the U.S.A."[63] Presumably the reference concerns Yogananda's sensational encounter with the 200 angry husbands of Miami, which had occurred some seven years prior, though it seems odd that this incident alone would have created such a long-lasting impression. The "bad press" was ultimately silenced by a close friend of Yogananda who had connections in journalism.

The unflattering publicity and organization-related disagreements were not the only unsavory aspects of Yogananda's return. His younger brother, Bishnu Charan Ghosh, had apparently inherited Yogananda's ambitious nature. During the fifteen years of Yogananda's American sojourn, Ghosh had made a name for himself as a prominent physical culturalist. Yogananda was quite impressed with this brother's establishment and even more impressed with the funding he had been able to secure to support his center. There was talk of collaboration. Ultimately, however, when Ghosh had arranged for Yogananda to demonstrate one of his most impressive yogic talents—stopping the heart—before a number of wealthy potential sponsors, things took a poor turn. Sailendra Bejoy Dasgupta, who served as Yogananda's secretary for the duration of the trip, recounts:

> Later, Bishnu Charan disappointedly said in a quiet tone of voice, "Mejda [Yogananda] ruined everything. He wasn't able to stop his heart from beating." However, nothing about this was ever brought out. During this time, the writer [Dasgupta] went one day to see Guru Maharaj [Sri Yukteswar] in Serampore. Although that particular event was never mentioned anywhere, it was known that Bishtu-da [Ghosh] had organized events for Swamiji [Yogananda] in many places, particularly in wealthy Marwari circles. After listening to everything, Gurudev [Sri Yukteswar] remained quiet for a while and then commented, "He [Yogananda] has a disease— where a ghoul comes and sits on his back. First there was Basu-ghoul [Dhirananda], and now Bishtu-ghoul [Ghosh] is sitting on his back.[64]

No joint venture between Yogananda and his brother ever materialized. Sri Yukteswar's attitude toward the prospect is generally reflective of the tension that characterized their reunion. Upon hearing about Yogananda's demonstrations of mental power in other contexts, Sri Yukteswar denounced the whole matter as "tricks" having nothing to do with spirituality. Dasgupta's account even hints that Yogananda's "Paramahansa" title may have been bestowed upon him by Sri Yukteswar as a sort of sarcastic joke, which Yogananda chose to interpret literally. In any case, relations between the two appear to have been strained at best.

The end of Yogananda's visit was marked by the death of Sri Yukteswar, who left his body while Yogananda was absent, having gone to the Kumbha Mela against his guru's request. Later accounts by Yogananda, including the entire chapter devoted to the event in his *Autobiography*, recount a vision of Sri Yukteswar one week after his passing in which he returned to Yogananda from the astral plane to disclose the secrets of the universe. A more immediate account, retold by Dasgupta, confirms Yogananda's vision but reveals a very different message:

> It is certain that the pain of not being able to fulfill Gurudev's last wishes gnawed at Yoganandaji from within; this is evidenced by Swamiji's desire that, before he left for America, he would go to each of the village-centers in Midnapore in which Gurudev had left his footprints. . . . The party reached Bombay. Preparatory activities for the journey were being conducted in the ship. Swamiji's heart was heavy-laden. As he was going to sleep at night in his hotel, suddenly, like a dream, he saw Sriyuktesvarji physically appear in his room. Yoganandaji looked at Gurudev's face

and said, "Why are you so disappointed?! Are you offended so much?!" Swamiji retold this statement to the writer [Dasgupta] later. . . . After this vision, Swamiji postponed his travel to America for the time being and returned with his assistants to Calcutta. It is true however that on New Year's Day—January 1, 1937, during the first public speech after he went back to America, Yoganandaji described the above-mentioned event as the resurrection of Sriyuktesvarji. A professional in the psychological sciences may say that the vision was a reflection of Swamiji's own pained state of mind.[65]

It is curious that Dasgupta, who has no qualms with attributing superpowers to anyone—including Yogananda—in his accounts, would conclude that Yogananda's vision of Sri Yukteswar had been nothing but a product of grief and imagination. Whatever the nature and content of this "revelation," however, his guru's passing had an undeniable effect on Yogananda. He became more introverted, immersing himself in organizational tasks, though any notions of working in collaboration with his brother's fitness center gradually faded away and eventually disappeared entirely.

Yogananda left India in 1936, never to return again. Despite more difficult times to come with Chowdhury's departure in 1939, Yogananda's American operation was prospering. By 1937 the SRF owned seventeen acres of land and was gearing up to begin a $400,000 building and improvement project, which included the building of a grand Golden Lotus Temple near Encinitas. The temple was erected on a hilltop overlooking the ocean, easily to be seen by motorists traveling on the Pacific Coast Highway. Unfortunately, the temple's picturesque location resulted in a majority of the construction sliding into the ocean in 1942. Perfection remained elusive.

Apotheosis and a Small Brown Spot

After Chowdhury's exit and the subsequent lawsuit, which lasted well into 1941, Yogananda's life appeared to take on a quieter tone. He never took on another close associate, though devoted disciples continued to flock to Mt. Washington, especially after the publication of Yogananda's magnum opus. The *Autobiography* was released in 1946, marking the only significantly publicized event of this final decade of the Swami's life.

Yogananda took his final *samādhi* on March 7, 1952. He died of an apparent heart attack while speaking at a dinner honoring Indian Ambassador Binay R. Sen at the Biltmore Hotel in Los Angeles. Yogananda was nearing the end of a short introductory address and, having proclaimed the importance of good relations between India and the United States, collapsed. Attempts to revive him by audience members and a promptly summoned ambulance crew proved unsuccessful. Close disciples claim that, in the preceding days, a change had come over the Master, and he had spoken as if to hint that he would soon be leaving them. Accounts of whether or not Yogananda finished the introductory address vary.

The condition of Yogananda's body has long served as a final testament to his superhuman status, especially among devotees. Excerpts from Yogananda's official mortuary report, issued by Forest Lawn Memorial Park, are included at the end of all SRF editions of Yogananda's *Autobiography*, attesting that "[t]he absence of any visual signs of decay in the dead body of Paramhansa Yogananda offers the most extraordinary case in our experience." Yogananda's body was embalmed twenty hours after death, at which point it had not begun to exhibit any signs of mold or desiccation. It was then interred twenty days later but remained under a heavy glass cover for the majority of that time.

It appears, however, that Forest Lawn Memorial Park's mortuary director may have been a bit over-enthusiastic in his affirmations of the extraordinary and unprecedented nature of Yogananda's lack of visible decomposition. A cursory investigation of these claims has been conducted by Leonard Angel,[66] who was able to ascertain that the uniqueness of the phenomenon had been greatly overstated. Angel's method generally consisted of picking out at random two licensed embalmers from the local Yellow Pages. Both contacts, who were credentialed professionals with many years of experience, confirmed that it was not at all unusual for a body to retain its appearance for over a month, especially given good conditions and a skilled embalmer. SRF reprints of the mortuary report generally exclude the paragraphs that refer to Yogananda's body being embalmed. An even more problematic omission is a pair of sentences in the report that even the otherwise unadulterated amazement of the mortuary director could not suppress: "On the late morning on March 26th, we observed a very slight, a barely noticeable change—the appearance on the tip of the nose of a brown spot, about one-fourth inch in diameter. This small faint spot indicated that the process of desiccation (drying up) might finally be starting."[67]

4

Yogi Calisthenics

*Password for March: "The Universe is mine. I am It." . . .
Having learned to decombobitate and concentrate yourself,
the next step is Meditation. Without concentration you can
do nothing, but concentration without meditation is profitless.
By meditation you devisualize and introspifficate the superior
or upper brain. Begin by short-circuiting your left leg by tying
around it a strip of red flannel, which polarizes your electrical
energy. Now place your chin in your left hand with your right
hand upon your solar plexus. In about half an hour you will
begin to feel the ether. The moment it comes stand upon your
left foot and swing with the right, like a pendulum, slowly at
first and gradually increasing to 75 per minute. Do this for
40 minutes then shift. While you are penduluming hold your
left hand at the small of your back and the right on top of your
head. You now have confluensillated the five rivers of life in
your solar plexus and are now meditating and sending out
vibrations of Love, Encouragement, and Happiness. To stop
vibrating, remove the red flannel bandage, cough three times,
and strike your right foot against the floor"*

—"HOME COURSE IN NEW THOUGHT. CONDUCTED BY
PANAMAHATMA MCGINNIS," *Chicago Daily Tribune*

IF THE YOGI is an instantiation of the human's destiny to become superhuman,
then it is inevitable that this process must begin with the concerns of the most
quotidian humanity. For Yogananda, as for his universalist predecessors, the figure of the Yogi embodied every human's potential to reach this (super)natural
goal. Consequently, his teaching often eschewed the esoteric and philosophical
for the mundane and practical. The legacy of Yogananda's lineage, carried on
in the West by the SRF, lies in the esoteric practice of Kriya Yoga, the goal of
which is nothing short of total enlightenment. However, Yogananda's success as

"the most spectacular swami in Los Angeles"[1] was generally grounded more in self-help than it was in full-blown self-realization. In the following chapter, we will examine the details of Yogananda's method and its connections with modern forms of physical yoga practice. By incorporating the familiar forms of European physical culture with yogic goals, Yogananda was among the first to establish the bridge between the esoteric techniques of premodern *hatha* yoga and the postural practice of today.

Yogananda's first address to the International Conference of Religious Liberals, subsequently published as his first book, *The Science of Religion* (1920), adheres quite closely to Vivekananda's brand of yoga, down to rehearsing the four-yoga model that the latter had propagated in the West.[2] However, whereas Vivekananda saw this popularization of Indian spirituality almost exclusively as a means of channeling prestige and, more important, funds back to his home country, Yogananda's eye was very much trained on the American continent itself. Whereas, as Carl T. Jackson has stated, for Vivekananda, "the idea of establishing Vedanta centers in the United States was an unanticipated result rather than the original intent of this Western trip,"[3] Yogananda, from the start, perceived his predecessor's success as a spiritual beacon to be a shining light of opportunity in its own right. Vivekananda had been an important, if at times begrudgingly envied, model to Yogananda in his early youth. Having set out to seek his yogic fortune in the New World, Yogananda no doubt clung to Vivekananda's example as a roadmap to success.

According to Wendell Thomas, whose *Hinduism Invades America* (1930) is the first scholarly treatment of Yogananda and was published during the heyday of the Swami's rising popularity, Yogananda's approach transformed drastically as he gained familiarity with his new environment. Thomas writes of Yogananda's initial lecture to the 1920 International Congress of Religious Liberals:

> Thinking this Congress wanted something theoretical and profoundly Hindu, the swami did not explain his educational methods or yoga technique, but spoke on "The Science of Religion," a work which had already been published in India, and was later elaborated and printed in book form in America. While in Boston, however, he learned something very practical. Coming into contact with various American cults such as Christian Science and New Thought, he began to admire their efficient methods of propaganda. At the same time, he was convinced that they were teaching only smatterings of the truth that Hinduism possessed as a whole. So he conceived the idea of combining his genuine Hindu message with American methods, and stayed in a new land to teach.[4]

However, in the thirty years since Vivekananda's US tour, the American public had been exposed to a far greater variety of phenomena that qualified as yoga.

Even Vivekananda's successors, like Swami Abhedananda, did not fully share his dismissal of superpowers and physical practice. In the same year that our Yogananda would arrive on American shores, a different Swami Yogananda was making waves in the New York medical community. Manibhai Haribhai Desai—who went by the title of Swami Yogananda during his brief visit to the United States between 1919 and 1923 and later became widely known in his native India as Shri Yogendra—performed not only *āsana*s but also superhuman feats such as inflating alternating lungs, altering the temperature of his extremities at will, and manipulating the electrical lights in the room and stopping his watch by means of electromagnetic energies emanating from his body.[5] Thus, immersion in the American scene demanded that our Yogananda acclimate to the spiritual climate of his market and it must have become quickly obvious to the newly arrived Swami that his audience was after more than just abstruse, if exotic, philosophy.

After his initial address in Boston, Yogananda continued to take any opportunity he could for speaking engagements in the Northeast. The end of 1920 found him, perhaps not surprisingly, a guest of Pierre Bernard, the infamous "Omnipotent Oom," who was by then a well-respected citizen and estate holder in Nyack, New York. Although the rumors of tantric rituals and late-night orgies had more or less died down, Bernard's Clarkstown Country Club was a regular stop for any Indian scholar or spiritual aspirant who came through the area. As Llwellyn Smith Jackson, a long-time disciple of Bernard better known as Cheerie, recalled, Yogananda

> stood out dramatically in his yellow robe, his very large brown eyes with long black lashes, his long raven-colored curls resting on his shoulders. . . . He lectured on yoga, ending the talk with a song, accompanied with an Indian instrument which he played. The song, "Oh, God, Beautiful" . . . he sang over and over, rolling his lustrous eyes lovingly and generously in the direction of the pretty girls watching him.[6]

On the subject of Yogananda's association with the man whom Robert Love, Bernard's biographer, identifies as the father of American *haṭha* yoga, Love goes so far as to claim that "Bernard and Yogananda respectfully parted ways after this visit for good reason: the Indian swami was uninterested in hatha yoga—disdained it, actually—and never taught it; Bernard placed hatha yoga at the center of a rapidly growing enterprise that was becoming more varied by the day."[7] While Love's characterization might be apt in the case of Vivekananda, Yogananda, as this chapter will duly show, held no marked disdain for *haṭha* yoga. He did regularly caution his disciples against tantra, his father's warnings after his youthful association with the red-eyed *sādhu* having apparently struck a nerve. So too would Yogananda have certainly disapproved of Bernard's advocacy of sexual rituals, despite later being haunted by accusations nearly identical to those that plagued the Omnipotent Oom at the height of his infamy. Still if, as Joseph Laycock has argued, Pierre Bernard is to be credited with "reforming the American perception of yoga from a scandalous practice associated with idolatry and perverse sexuality into a wholesome system of fitness,"[8] such a claim must be taken with a race-tinged grain of salt. After all, no matter how many times Bernard got arrested for abducting and corrupting impressionable young ladies, his whiteness allowed him a prestige with which even the most exotically alluring Indian Swami was hard-pressed to contend. To his credit, Yogananda appeared to take Bernard's example to heart in more ways than one. He too recognized that the best way to make a potentially scandalous practice appealing to white American elites was to stage it in a country club.

Love's claim regarding Yogananda's disinterest in and disdain for *hatha* yoga, however, is simply untrue. In fact, for lack of explicit information regarding what it was that Bernard in fact learned from his mysterious guru, Sylvais Hamati, Yogananda might have been practicing a more "authentic"[9] form of *hatha* yoga than Bernard himself. On the other hand, given the working model with which Yogananda arrived on American shores, it is not difficult to believe that his self-presentation at Bernard's club might have given the impression of a Vivekananda-like disregard for physical practice. It is also not unlikely that it was at Bernard's oasis of alternative spirituality blended with physical culture that Yogananda stumbled upon a far more current vision of what his prospective audience was truly interested in.

Through the course of the next three decades, Yogananda would mold himself and his message into a sleek modern system of holistic spirituality best described by the title of the periodical through which he would disseminate it, beginning in 1925: *East-West.* The wide-ranging yet practically topical scope of the rising Swami's agenda is aptly illustrated by the publication's second issue,[10] the contents of which feature a detailed exposé on the Tagua fern, dental care tips, a blurb on the Sikh Guru Nanak, a list of distinguished vegetarians ranging from Hesiod to General William Booth, an essay by Mohandas Gandhi on nationalism, and an essay by Yogananda on issues of American citizenship legislation. The latter essay treats specifically the case of Bhagat Singh Thind, whom Yogananda erroneously identifies as Hindu, and goes so far as to name senators serving on the federal Immigration Committee and encourages readers to write in protest of the exclusionary law. Later issues continue in this eclectic style, featuring a bricolage of poetry, encyclopedia-like articles on Sufism and Zen Buddhism, socially and politically engaged pieces by Yogananda on subjects from racist yellow journalism to the labor laws, explanations of the relationship between Yogoda and Christian Science, and excerpts from Ralph Waldo Trine's *In Tune with the Infinite* (1897).

Above all, Yogananda learned his audience and he learned them well. His ongoing efforts to remain relevant and pragmatic while simultaneously weaving in a distinct spiritual agenda would come to bear fruit as his popularity soared. The cornerstone of his appeal, along with his practical worldliness and raw charisma, was a reimagined version of yogic practice that was distinctly physical in nature. In a process that appears to have begun while he was still in India, Yogananda stripped the ritual practice of Kriya Yoga to its barest functional bones and reframed it in a context of therapeutic calisthenics coupled with a mind cure ideology. This body of teachings, which he would call Yogoda,[11] bears no resemblance to and yet at the same time is almost identical with modern forms of physical yogic practice. The former point accounts for the reason that Yogananda is uniformly overlooked in studies of the pedigree of postural yoga in America. His Yogoda Energization Exercises look nothing like either traditional or modern yoga *āsana*s. However, the functional role of his exercises is in total alignment with the use of *āsana*s in modern postural yoga insomuch as they are geared at conditioning the body, promoting health, and possibly preparing one for meditation.

There is a more specific point to be made here about the role and formation of postural practice in the Indian and especially transnational yoga of the early twentieth century. As Mark Singleton has thoroughly illustrated, *āsana* was during this time a tenuous and non-delineated component of yoga practice. The modern obsession with *āsana* practice emerged in part out of the complex interplay of nationalistic "muscular Hinduism," with its focus on man-building through physical culture, and the medicalizing efforts of figures like Swami Kuvalyananda.[12] On the other side of the world, the Western preoccupation with harmonial fitness offered a continually friendly port of call for the process of cross-cultural exchange that has lent modern postural yoga its current form. The bodily expressions we now refer to uniformly as *āsana*s, thus endowing them with a "traditional" Indian pedigree, hail from origins as diverse as medieval *haṭha* yogic manuals, regional Indian wrestling exercises, British military calisthenics, and Swedish gymnastics. It would be reasonable to assume that in Yogananda's time his Energization Exercises might not have seemed any more or less like "yoga poses" than some of the positions and movements to which that title is accorded today without a second thought.

And yet Yogananda's system is rarely if ever mentioned in overviews of American yogic practice. The only immediately evident explanation is that Yogananda himself never referred to his exercises as *āsana*s, nor has the SRF ever pushed for such an identification. Since scholarship on modern postural yoga has hit its stride only over the last decade, in a context in which the postural canon of modern yoga has more or less been formalized through print media and decades of popular practice, the oversight is not surprising. However, in light of Singleton's findings, Yogananda's system merits full inclusion under the umbrella of modern postural yoga, at least for taxonomic purposes.

Yogoda, a title that has now been subsumed into the modified version of Kriya Yoga espoused by the SRF, is a masterful adaptation of a traditional Indian tantric and *haṭha* yogic techniques into a Western register of harmonial wellness. Moreover, it is a prime example of what Alter refers to as a marriage of the *haṭha* yogic "perfection of the body" to the modern cosmetic fitness model[13] that has come to characterize the practice of modern postural yoga. Yogananda's integration of European physical culture with Indian *haṭha* yogic ideology signals an important step in the complex transition not only into a model of yoga as fitness but fitness as ritual spirituality.

Yogi Gymnastics and Progressive Era Health Culture

Yogoda arose in a context where the methods of Yogis—real or purported— were already becoming embedded in the simmering blend of Progressive Era alternative spirituality, health consciousness, sexual politics, and other heralds of modernism. Yogananda's target demographic was the same high society that sustained Vivekananda's legacy of Vedanta Society centers and rocketed esotericist playboys like Bernard to dazzling infamy. As we saw in chapter 1 through the testimony presented over Sara Bull's involvement with the aforementioned organization, Americans were slowly becoming exposed to the basic hallmarks of yoga methodology: breathing exercises, energy manipulation, and meditative techniques. Furthermore, while Vivekananda did not teach postural practice, the publications of subsequent Vedanta Society leaders indicate that basic *āsana*s were most likely part of the curriculum. Then, of course, there was the "weird, fantastic form of calisthenics" reportedly practiced at Pierre Bernard's Clarkstown Country Club.

The momentum that caused postural yoga practice to overtake Vivekananda's more mystically inclined vision, even within his own organization, had been building for decades. Nineteenth-century Spiritualist activists advocated for dress reform, gymnastics, temperance, vegetarianism, and water cure not only to invigorate the bodies of men but to free the bodies of women from the shackles of Victorian feminine frailty.[14] Such countercultural trends found their counterbalance in the Evangelical Muscular Christianity movement, which depicted strength, aggression, and muscularity as not just masculine but pious traits.[15]

Physical culture, even without any spiritual trappings, was on the rise through-out the second half of the nineteenth century as a response to the increasingly sedentary lifestyles of the post-Industrial middle and upper classes. Such move-ments were especially popular in England, Germany, and the United States. Nevertheless, grounded in the legacy of Mesmerism and other esoterically linked ideologies, from German Lebensreform[16] to American mind cure, physical cul-ture, naturopathy, and alternative spirituality often went hand-in-hand.

The epigraph that opens this chapter, a satirical blurb published by the *Chicago Daily Tribune* in 1902, illustrates that at the very outset of the twentieth century physical exercises were already a part of the general cultural conflation of New Thought mind cure, metaphysical ideology, and health consciousness. Although his formal publication on the topic, *Hatha Yoga or the Yogi Philosophy of Physical Well-Being*, would not be released until 1904, the subject of the satire is most likely Yogi Ramacharaka, also known as William Walker Atkinson. Atkinson was active on Chicago's New Thought scene at the time and it is not unlikely that he might have propagated the book's contents before its publication. However, despite its title, there is very little yoga or indeed anything else of Indian origin in the book's pages. It is largely an overview of contemporary understandings of the human health, diet, and other related topics with sections devoted to basic breathing exercises and some minor calisthenics. It is the latter section that is of most importance to us as it contains chiefly the exact type of pendular arm and leg exercises that the *Tribune* finds so amusing. However, such exercises, typical of Euro-American physical culture at the time, are also extremely similar to those later promoted by Yogananda.

Unlike Yogananda, Atkinson's knowledge of Indian systems of thought was cursory at best, as evidenced by his frequent representation of New Thought and other Western esoteric principles under the guise of ancient yogic truth. He would have had basic access to more traditional versions of *haṭha* yoga— Abhedananda's *How to Be a Yogi* (1902) contains not only more accurate repre-sentations of the premises of this system but description of several recognizable yogic *āsana*s. However, Ramacharaka's book puts forth an explicit explanation for the absence of such forms that both legitimates his method and underhandedly discredits his competitor, who freely acknowledges that *haṭha* yogis are not only after physical health but bona fide superpowers. Appealing to a lingering Western Romanticism, Ramacharaka specifies that real "Hatha Yoga" aspires to no more than to return man to the proper state of nature. He further explains that the reason this branch of yoga has heretofore been dismissed is due to the actions of Indian pretenders—"a horde of mendicants of the lower fakir class, who pose as Hatha Yogis . . . acquiring the ability to perform certain abnormal 'tricks' which they exhibit to amuse and entertain (or disgust) Western travelers."[17] He then goes on to liken these performers to Western "freaks" and invoke other popular images of Indian Yogis as dirty and misshapen ascetics, whose abilities, while curious, do not represent anything "which is of the slightest interest to the man or woman seeking to maintain a healthy, normal, natural body." Indeed, the author reveals that he does know the traditional purview of *haṭha* yoga by specifying that his is not *that* kind of book. It would not "tell you how to assume seventy-four types of postures, nor how to draw linen through the intestines for the purpose of cleaning them (contrast this with nature's plans) or how to stop the heart's beating, or to perform tricks with your internal apparatus." It strives only toward "making man a healthy being—not to make a 'freak' of him."[18]

Such protestations took aim at an audience that wanted the Oriental mystique and authority of yoga without having to embrace the realities of Indian Yogis or their practices. Their tastes were exotic, but not *too* exotic. This was an audience not quite prepared for the Vedanta Society's hygienic methods—the intestinal cleansing technique (*dhauti*) referenced by Ramacharaka is a traditional practice in premodern *haṭha* yoga and is explicitly cited in Abhedananda's book— nor for the "fantastic contortions" taught by Bernard.

However, in 1920, about a year after the *Los Angeles Times* made the above evaluation of Bernard's operation and a few months before Yogananda would arrive in Boston, the *Chicago Daily Tribune* ran an edition of its society section, penned by a Mme. X, titled "Gymnastics after Dinner Mark True Follower of Yogi."[19] The column, which eventually meanders into topics such as new open air dance locales, fundraising for the Girl Scouts, and a burdensome tax on antiques, begins with the following:

> Are you a Yogi? Have you a real Yogi mat, thickly wadded, and with big Thibetan tassels at the corners to hold it down? And do you spread it out in your drawing room after dinner, and, with your guests, as Yogi as yourself, do you thereon turn somersaults, bend your back until your head touches your heels, and indulge in various other supple and symbolic contortions which manifest the coordination of the body and soul?
>
> If not, you are not the very highest height of fashion in the east. I don't mean the remote east, where the Yogis are supposed to hang out, but that nearer and dearer east, a little beyond the sunrise, whence come so many of our cheerful follies. . . . You can, of course, be a quiet yogi, and sit on the floor, with your head on your knees, your arms clasped around your shins, your eyes closed, your whole being absorbed in contemplation of the infinite and eternal. But for a dinner party this is not so social a form of Yogiism as the other, though after some sumptuous feasts it would be a

great relief to be able to withdraw into some such state of complete mental and bodily torpor.[20]

Here, we see an emerging distinction in the popular understanding of yoga, or "Yogiism," and the dynamic form of yogic gymnastics appears to be winning out, even if superficially, over the purely meditative mysticism that characterized the initial positive conceptions of Yogis in the West. We also see that tolerance for more extreme postural forms appears to be increasing, at least among those who, as Andrea Jain has described them "could afford, both financially and socially, to be eccentric."[21] The relationship between these two types of yoga, one distinctly spiritual and the other ostentatiously physical, remained ambiguous.

Yogananda consistently maintained a balance between the more esoteric aspects of *haṭha* yoga and popularizing versions that relied on more familiar physical practices. Especially in his early days in the United States, he would occasionally personally demonstrate advanced *āsanas*—such as balancing on his hands while in a full lotus seat (*utthita padmāsana*)—as proof of the effectiveness of his method of willful muscle control. However, he was careful to contextualize such displays by incorporating them into a holistic system of Western-friendly bodily and mental health. This is especially evident in Yogoda's reliance on European calisthenics rather than yogic *āsanas*. While more advanced and traditional techniques, including a full if modified version of Kriya Yoga, were available to committed disciples, he was careful to avoid anything that could be perceived as "freakish" in his more publicly available materials. Nevertheless, although Yogananda's system resembles Ramacharaka's purely-European fitness program masquerading as yoga, it is novel and unique in its careful integration of *haṭha* yogic logic and methodology.

Adaptations of Kriya Yoga

Yogananda did not altogether abandon the distinctly Indian *haṭha* yogic techniques of Kriya Yoga. However, because Kriya Yoga requires initiation and calls for committed and sustained practice, it was not particularly practical as a source of material for public lectures and demonstrations. The SRF continues to initiate students into the technique via the series of lessons that Yogananda composed and left behind. Because Yogananda decreed himself to be the last in the line of Kriya Yoga gurus—at least in the West, since presumably the swamis in Sri Yukteswar's continuing lineage as well as other remaining disciples of Lahiri Mahasaya might very well be considered gurus in their own right—the written lessons, after the Sikh fashion, have become guru in his stead.

Although *kriyā*s (here best translated as "exercises") may incorporate *āsana*s, they are generally composed of several different elements and may therefore be quite complex as the following list will demonstrate. The number of *kriyā*s ranges anywhere from 108 to 7 to 4. Most sources agree, however, that this discrepancy is more a matter of variously formalized subdivisions than actual additional practices. Yogananda's *Autobiography* states that Lahiri Mahasaya distilled the complex practice passed on to him by Babaji into four essential stages. This general schema seems to be confirmed by the writings of others from his lineage. For instance, Satyeswarananda produces a total of eleven "original Kriyas" by listing each step of the initial stage separately and individually enumerating four different *omkāra* (*om*-making) *kriyā*s, whereas Satyananda and Dasgupta cite four, with possible subsequent levels that are attained through the practitioner's own intuition and without the formal aid of a guru. Generally, the four stages of the original practice can be broken up as follows:

(1) "first *kriyā*"

    a. *mahāmudrā* (great seal): *prāṇāyāma* (breath control) is coupled with a *haṭha* yogic exercise resembling *paścimottānāsana* (a seated forward bend).

    b. *nābhi mudrā* (navel seal): a hand seal is applied to the third *cakra* (navel) in several ways and the *om* syllable is chanted.

    c. *tālavya kriyā* (palatal exercise): a stretching of the lingual frenulum that is practiced as a preparatory technique for the eventual performance of *khecarī mudrā*, where the tongue reaches into the nasal cavity.[22]

    d. "*kriyā* proper": *prāṇāyāma* performed with a seed *mantra*, generally repeated many times and serving a purifying function akin to a tantric *bhūta-śuddhi* (purification of the material body).

    e. *yoni mudrā* (source seal):[23] a hand seal is used to close off the sense organs of the face such that the body's subtle light is perceived in the third eye and the divine sound begins to emerge. Yogananda refers to this technique as "Jyoti Mudra" ("Light Seal").

(2) *omkāra kriyā* (*om*-making exercise): a multi-level practice that involves imposition of *mantra* syllables and *cakra* (energy center) visualization coupled with *prāṇāyāma*, including the *thokar* ("pecking") technique, which incorporates head movements.[24]

(3) *brahmayoni mudrā*: similar in technique to the *omkāra kriyā*s,[25] with the goal being to establish the *praṇava* sound (the syllable *om*) fully in the *brahmayoni* (third eye).

(4) *pūrṇa kriyā* (full exercise): relies on energy channeling techniques learned in the *omkāra kriyā*s, but dispenses with *mantra* practice, as the divine inner

sound arises naturally at this stage.[26] The practitioner uses advanced breathing techniques to consecutively raise and lower energy in order to break through the *mūlādhāra granthi* (root knot) and release the *kuṇḍalinī*, or the latent spiritual energy coiled at the base of the spine.

As should be evident from the above, Kriya Yoga is a fairly standard form of tantric *haṭha* yoga. Through the various steps of the practice, the adept's body is perfected into a powerful battery (to use Yogananda's terminology) of divine energy. However, because the practice still largely relies on oral transmission from guru to disciple, details about the specific techniques are difficult to ascertain. Moreover, what written accounts do exist are generally vague and not particularly systematic in their nomenclature and classifications. Although there is general consensus on the elements of the first *kriyā*, the order of the exercises may be modified, some may be repeated, and some eliminated. For instance, Yogananda is frequently criticized for excluding the practice of *khecarī mudrā*. This is not altogether true, as some disciples of Yogananda (most notably Kriyananda) report being taught *khecarī*, or at the very least hearing him speak about it. However, Yogananda evidently did eliminate the practice as a mandatory prerequisite for advancement to initiation into the second *kriyā*. After the first stage, subsequent *kriyās* appear to build on the *oṃkāra* technique of subtle pneumatics as the practitioner progressively learns to channel his *prāṇa* through the body's energy centers (*cakras*). However, the number of distinct *kriyās* varies among the different accounts, as do their divisions. In adapting this four-stage system, Yogananda (and the SRF) dispenses with the nomenclature altogether and simply refers to the *kriyās* numerically as first, second, and so on.

Although the particulars are difficult to discern due to the persistent esotericism of the SRF's core teachings, it appears that Yogananda kept the basic structure of Kriya Yoga practice more or less intact for the Westerners whom he initiated. As noted above, he dispensed with *khecarī mudrā* as a requirement, recommending it only to select disciples, as he thought that the technique's difficulty and general strangeness would not win much popularity with a Western audience. *Nābhi mudrā* evidently met with a similar fate. On the whole, Yogananda made a number of changes to the first *kriyā* in terms of form and required content—and presumably to the subsequent *kriyās* as well, though such differences in technique become increasingly difficult to recognize for the uninitiated. These changes were geared at rendering the practice more approachable for his American disciples. Most visibly, the practitioner was migrated from his traditional *padmāsana* (cross-legged lotus seat) to sit upright in a straight-backed chair. As might be expected, members of Yogananda's lineage generally did not take kindly to these modifications with some, like Satyeswarananda, expressing great consternation over how the body is to levitate during the final stages of Kriya practice if the legs are left dangling free.

In addition to the excisions and modifications, Yogananda also made some additions to his version of the Kriya Yoga practice. Most notable are the thirty-seven Energization Exercises that form the backbone of his Yogoda method, as well as the Hong-Saw and Om meditation techniques. The latter two are actually not so much Yogananda's own additions as they are simplified transpositions of techniques appearing elsewhere in the practice. Hong-Saw is an anglicization of the "ham-sa"[27] mantra reportedly taught by Sri Yukteswar. Both techniques are geared toward introducing the practitioner to basic concentration and breath control.

Charging the Body Battery: The Origins of Yogoda

Although this fact is seldom emphasized by current insider and scholarly accounts alike, Yogananda exhibited an early interest in physical culture on par with any of the typically cited giants of postural yoga. In his youth Yogananda was an avid athlete who excelled in running, wrestling, and soccer. He also regularly trained with weights. As spiritual pursuits began to consume more of Yogananda's time, he left behind the distracting realm of team and competitive sports. However, physical culture would become a permanent fixture of his work, ultimately culminating in the Energization Exercises that are taught by the SRF to this day. These exercises, consisting largely of gentle calisthenics and muscle control through interchanging tension and relaxation, were originally introduced as part of Yogananda's Yogoda system, which constituted a core aspect of his marketed teaching during the initial decade after his arrival to the United States.

The system was first implemented at Yogananda's school for young boys at Ranchi, where he incorporated it into a broader curriculum of general education. Despite the modern attitude articulated by Yogananda's devotees and expressed in the materials of the SRF and Ananda—namely, that these teachings stem from ancient yogic truths—the Energization Exercises in fact appear to have a less exotic origin. Yogananda himself states that the Yogoda method was "discovered" by him in 1916,[28] the same year as the founding of his school. The details of this discovery are illuminated by Satyananda's account, which specifies the following:

> About a year before the founding of the school, a book written by a German physical culturalist named Miller came into Yoganandaji's hands.

He was enthused and excited upon reading in the book about muscle-building through mental power. Seeing me, he said, "I have found exactly what I was looking for." This book had greatly helped in systematizing the "Yogoda" method. Swamiji had experienced that power could be gathered via the inexhaustible internal will of human beings, by which, different muscles could be controlled and strengthened; without using tools or machines, the body could be made strong and powerful by natural techniques [mind and body] alone. . . . The bodybuilding education of Yoganandaji's youngest brother—now the eminent physical culturalist Sri Bishnu Charan Ghosh—actually began here. Of course, later on [Sri Bishnu Charan Ghosh] received inspiration from the famous physical culturalist Chittun and other great athletes.[29]

Unfortunately, no Miller appears to exist among the ranks of well-known German physical culturalists of the time who would fit the required qualifications. The birth name of Eugen Sandow, German icon of the turn-of-the-century Ironman movement, was Friedrich Wilhelm Müller. However, Sandow never published anything under that name, and in any case his style was almost exclusively focused on exercises with dumbbells rather than mental power. A better candidate might be Danish physical culturalist, Jørgen Peter Müller, whose 1904 work, *Mit System* (*My System*), was translated into twenty-five different languages.[30]

Upon close examination, Müller's repertoire of exercises appears to resemble to a remarkable extent the exercises prescribed by Yogananda in the early pamphlets detailing his Yogoda method. For instance, the two systems include torso-rotation exercises that are virtually identical in practice, with the exception of the positioning of the arms (see figs. 4.1 and 4.2). Generally speaking, though the ordering is different, Yogananda's system is based on a series of pendular and rotational moves applied to the torso, arms, and legs that are quite similar if not identical to Müller's. Despite these structural points of convergence, however, the two systems ultimately appear different in focus and overall methodology. Müller's system does place extensive emphasis on coordinating breath with movement but ultimately does not concern itself much with muscular control. Rather, it cultivates flexibility and "looseness" in the muscles and joints, even relying on momentum where necessary. Yogananda's system, on the other hand, is based on a conscious and willful flexing and relaxing of isolated muscles even in the midst of sustained movement. A similar emphasis can be found in other body-building manuals of the day, which focus on flexing isolated muscle groups in order to develop control and tone. Even more telling, if one is looking to attribute influence, is Müller's complete lack of concern with the role of the mind in any of his work. Thus, though there are enough points of convergence to suggest that

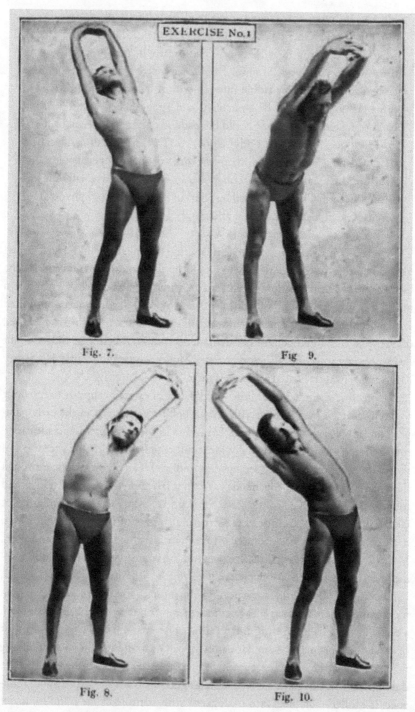

FIGURE 4.1 Müller's "Slow Trunk Circling Exercise" from his *My System* (1904)

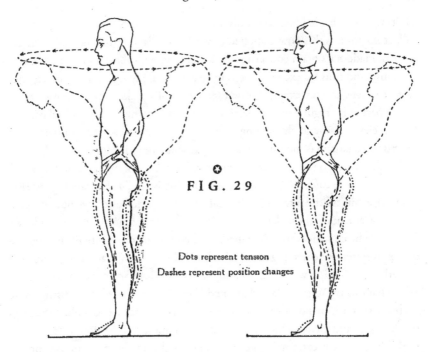

FIG. 29

Dots represent tension
Dashes represent position changes

FIGURE 4.2 Yogananda's "Exercise for Waist" from his *Yogoda or Tissue-Will System of Physical Perfection* (1925)

Yogananda was familiar with Müller's work, and possibly modeled many of the Energization Exercises on its anatomical forms, *Mit System* is most likely not the "book about muscle-building through mental power" to which Satyananda refers.

It would not be unreasonable to assume that Yogananda owned more than a single book. Singleton has suggested that the Yogoda system owes much to New Thought, specifically the work of Jules Payot and Frank Channing Haddock.[31] Although Yogananda must certainly have adopted much from New Thought during his lengthy sojourn in the United States, Satyananda's account confirms that he was in fact implementing the principles of mental body-building in India before he was immersed in the New Thought scene in any significant way, as such materials were at this time only beginning to filter into India. Haddock's *Power of the Will* was first published in 1907, so it is not impossible that Yogananda might have secured a copy.

Haddock's work does include a few lightly calisthenic exercises that resemble some of the leg and arm swinging that one finds in Müller's book. However, the similarities between the exercises prescribed by Yogananda and by Müller are far more numerous, and thus it makes little sense to assume that Yogananda would have appropriated them from Haddock rather than from the original source. In addition, though Haddock certainly puts a marked emphasis on the power of will, at no point is this power applied toward muscular control and development as such. Haddock's main concern is conscious and willful movement in the general sense, and thus his exercises focus primarily on applying mindfulness to one's every movement—for example, one exercise entails picking up a book—rather than a particular regime of gymnastics. Furthermore, the flexing and relaxing of the muscles as a way of channeling energy through the power of will that are so central to Yogananda's method are entirely absent from Haddock's work.

With respect to the possible influence of Payot's work on Yogananda, Payot's *L'Éducation de la volonté* (1893, translated into English as *The Education of the Will* in 1909), exhibits little interest in physical culture beyond basic hygiene and a general endorsement of "muscular exercise." In the absence of more concrete evidence, it can only be concluded that Yogananda relied on one or—more likely—several books to systematize his Yogoda method. It is likely that Jørgen Peter Müller is indeed the "Miller" to whom Satyananda refers, but that Satyananda was mistaken as to what exactly Yogananda had gleaned from the man's work. It is furthermore probable that Yogananda also came across one or more sources detailing the ways in which will and mental power can be applied to muscular development.

Ultimately, it is extremely likely Yogananda also made some innovations of his own, possibly including the integration of muscular tension and relaxation with principles of will and energy-manipulation. Singleton is probably correct to point out the influence of Payot and Haddock on Yogananda's work in the larger sense. It seems likely that they might well have been the sources of Yogananda's preoccupation with the language of will. In Haddock's work, especially, we find a spiritualized will that is described as an "energy," thereby likening the mind to an "electric battery."[32] Yogananda appears to have expanded on this notion with his concept of the "body battery" that yokes the body and mind into a single energetic continuum. Here, Yogananda's Indian roots in tantric energetics yield something more integrated than Haddock's exercises in mindfulness. The Energization Exercises of Yogoda not only train and hone the power of the will but actively effect a beneficial flow of energy through the body. Haddock's exercises—calisthenic or otherwise—are a means to an end, the end being a powerful and controlled will. Yogananda's Energization Exercises are a small end in themselves insofar as they effect the flow of energy represented by the will. Thus, the relationship between physical (energetic) practice and psycho-spiritual development becomes reciprocal, as it would be in *haṭha* yogic traditions. From this perspective, Yogananda's system represents a transformation of the psycho-centric practices of Western metaphysical mind cure as represented by Payot and Haddock and a step toward the embodied psychosomatic therapy represented by modern postural yoga.

Yogananda clearly began developing some of these ideas while still in India at the Ranchi school. However, this was not the message that he first intended to bring to America, as evidenced by his inaugural address in Boston. Even if Yogananda was aware of New Thought principles prior to his arrival in the United States, it is evident that he was not anticipating the extent to which they held sway over his new audience. The continued development of Yogoda signals a realization on Yogananda's part that practical yoga, as embodied in his own lineage, held much greater potential than the neo-Vedāntin philosophy espoused by Vivekananda. In this sense, Yogananda's ritual training and initiation into a formalized *sādhana* gave him a distinct edge over his predecessor and most of his contemporaries. While it would not have been practical or, from a traditional viewpoint, ethical to market Kriya Yoga to the mass public, its ritual complex proved to be a rich resource for Yogananda's metaphysical synthesis.

*A Note on Ā*sana *Practice*

Although the SRF's iteration of Kriya Yoga remains fundamentally *haṭha* yogic in character, one cannot help but note the marked absence of *āsana*s from its repertoire. A close look at Yogananda's biographical sources quickly illustrates that he was no stranger to physical culture, yet he is nowhere explicitly described as practicing or having any training in *āsana*s. This remains true until one turns to the somewhat adjacent tradition of Yogananda's youngest bother Bishnu Ghosh, who would go on to become a major figure in the postural yoga landscape. It also bears noting that Ghosh, whose yoga is precisely what we think of when referring to postural practice today, traces his lineage directly through his older brother. Although we have few details from Ghosh himself, his descendants and disciples claim it was during his time at Yogananda's Ranchi school that he learned the eighty-four classical *āsana*s that would later be distilled into the popular Bikram Yoga sequence and are still taught in full as Bikram Choudhury's "advanced class." These *āsana*s apparently constituted an integral part of Yogananda's Yogoda method at the time.[33]

This suggests that the substitution of *āsana*s with the considerably more basic and Westerner-friendly Energization Exercises was simply another facet of Yogananda's process of adaptation. He does note in his *Autobiography* that the boys at his Ranchi school, as the first to be subjected to the Yogoda regimen, were able to "sit in perfect poise in difficult body postures."[34] Given that no aspect of the Energization Exercises can be considered objectively "difficult," it is possible that the system of physical development practiced at Ranchi was in fact something more akin to Ghosh's eighty-four posture sequence than to the basic calisthenics that would inherit this function. Because the Indian branch of the SRF, still officially known as the Yogoda Satsanga Society (YSS), has been under Western management since Yogananda's passing (with no small amount of legal wrangling), its teachings reflect the version of Kriya Yoga, along with its Energization Exercises, propagated by Yogananda in America. No *āsana* practice is taught at the modern-day Ranchi school, though it suggestively specifies that "Paramahansa Yogananda encouraged their practice as very beneficial."[35]

However, a closer look at the offshoots of the SRF demonstrates that not only was Yogananda very much aware of *āsana* practice but that he taught it in the United States. Examining the offerings of the SRF's most prominent splinter group, Kriyananda's Ananda Church of Self Realization (operating as Ananda Sangha worldwide), one quickly notices the presence of postural practice as part of the prescribed method. Kriyananda has been emphatic about preserving Yogananda's original message, even going so far as to release an alternate version of the *Autobiography*, presented as it was first printed in 1946 before the SRF introduced a long series of edits that continued well past Yogananda's death. If Kriyananda's ostensible devotion to Yogananda's legacy is not enough to establish the origins of his postural offerings, a comparative analysis of the *āsanas* presented in Kriyananda's *Yoga Postures for Higher Awareness* (1967) illustrates a remarkable level of consistency with Ghosh's full sequence. Particular *āsanas*, such as *śaśaṅgāsana* ("Rabbit Pose"), and distinctive variations on other common postures are, to the best of my knowledge, unique to Ghosh's lineage in contemporary yoga practice and particularly serve to distinguish its variations from the more common Mysore style that originates from disciples of Tirumalai Krishnamacarya.

One is left to assume, then, that Yogananda treated *āsana* practice much as he treated other more advanced *haṭha* yogic techniques like *khecarī mudrā*. Disciples who claim he did not teach *āsana*s were simply not in the inner circle that Yogananda had deemed worthy or capable of such practices. Indeed, non-SRF-affiliated teachers of Yogananda's legacy maintain that this was precisely the case and that Yogananda instructed select male disciples in *āsana* practice and encouraged them to maintain it "if they felt it beneficial." Interestingly though perhaps not surprisingly, no such instruction was extended to female disciples.[36] Several photographs substantiate such claims, showing Yogananda instructing groups of disciples in relatively advanced poses, such as *śīrṣāsana* (headstand) and *mayūrāsana* (peacock pose). Other proponents of Kriya Yoga, who trace their lineage through Lahiri Mahasaya or Sri Yukteswar in ways that sometimes circumvent Yogananda altogether, likewise make references to the practice of "Hatha" (by which they almost certainly mean *āsana*) as a complement to the *kriyās*, which suggests that postural practice was involved in the original Indian forms of Kriya Yoga.

It is thus possible that Ghosh's tradition is the second half of the lineage currently represented by the SRF. It remains unclear what precisely happened in 1916. If Yogananda had indeed been teaching *āsana*s at the Ranchi school, he would have begun his own practice at a much earlier age. Given Yogananda's athleticism and spiritual promiscuousness, this would not be surprising. Consequently, the "discovery" of 1916 was likely one of theory rather than of technique. Immersing himself in European physical culture and its mind cure and will-centric corollaries, Yogananda must have made connections with the logics of energy underlying *haṭha* yoga. The specificities of physical form differed, but the methods and goals were ultimately comparable if not identical. Because *āsana*s as yet enjoyed no significant popularity and therefore held little cultural capital in the United States, it is not surprising that Yogananda made no effort to co-opt *āsana* forms or terminology into his Energization Exercises, choosing instead to adapt the physical conditioning to his Western audiences by relying on more familiar forms.[37] Had things been otherwise, the SRF might have found itself in a much different position in relation to the mainstream of modern American yoga.

Most fascinating, especially given the complete exclusion of this form of physical practice from the modern canon of *āsana*s, is the widespread nature of the Energization Exercises among Yogananda's contemporaries and competitors. Although largely ignoring the likely influences on Yogananda's method, Singleton has drawn connections between Müller's System and the teachings of at least two other "West Coast Yogis," namely Yogi Wassan and Yogi Hari Rama, whose published manuals contain illustrations of nearly identical exercises.[38] One possible conclusion—generally drawn by Singleton—is that the popularity of Müller's regimen and its offshoots, which yielded the "generic, ubiquitous illustrations of the kind seen in 1920s Western physical culture manuals,"[39] was not lost on the upstart Yogis of the same time period. However, if we consider the fact that Yogananda may have been using this same style of physical practice in India as early as 1916, as well as the fact that the publication of Yogananda's Yogoda pamphlets predates Wassan's and Hari Rama's versions, it could be argued that Yogananda had a much more pronounced influence on American physical yoga practice than previously supposed. There is, of course, no sure way of determining who copied whom. One possible hint lies in the naming of Wassan's "Soroda" system, which after all sounds suspiciously like "Yogoda." Granted, none of these systems appears to have achieved sufficient authority to sway what counts as "yoga" in the twenty-first century. One nevertheless wonders how the landscape of today's postural practice might look if Yogananda had chosen to refer to his Energization Exercises as *āsana*s.

Unlike Wassan and Hari Rama, whose legacies are preserved only through their largely out-of-print publications, Yogananda was ultimately able to secure an impressive organizational platform for his teachings. However, much of Yogananda's marketing genius lay in his ability to convey his material in a manner both relevant and accessible to his audience. Within the first three years of his sojourn in the United States, Yogananda's message appears to have transformed from the type of high-brow philosophical model established by Vivekananda to a more practically minded, embodied practice. However, when this shift occurred, it is not the complex tantric practice of Kriya Yoga that was allotted center stage, but rather the increasingly harmonially influenced system of Yogoda.

Yogoda on the Western Metaphysical Stage

Even in its simplified form, Kriya Yoga would have been on the fringes of the mainstream Western metaphysical spirituality. Its general principles of energy manipulation would not have been altogether unrecognizable, but the complex ritual aspect was rather foreign even to Americans versed in traditions such as Theosophy and New Thought. Based on the locations of Yogananda's early lectures in the Boston area, it appears that he circulated primarily in Unitarian communities, which were then heavily dominated by strains of New Thought. The Boston Brahmins, already steeped in the heritage of Transcendentalism, were quite amenable to Yogananda's vision. Although Christian Science has had a historically problematic relationship with Asian religions,[40] the more diffuse ideology of the New Thought movement freely incorporated Asian metaphysical concepts. Authors like Haddock, while not explicitly affiliated with New Thought, espoused ideologies that fell into the even broader and more amorphous category of mind cure.

The positive affirmation techniques employed by Haddock and co-opted by Yogananda, were popularized by Phineas P. Quimby, the first to incorporate Mesmeric hypnotism into a larger complex of holistic mental healing, and by Warren Felt Evans, Quimby's student and perhaps the most prolific of the early New Thought authors. Boston in particular was seen as an epicenter of confluence for all those tributaries of the modern New Age movement that ultimately focus on what Paul Heelas has identified as "Self-spirituality," or the divinization of the human self.[41] Yogananda was speaking to an audience already prepared by New Thought author Ralph Waldo Trine's claims, in his wildly popular *In Tune with the Infinite* (1907), that "when we come to the realization of the fact that we are God-men, then again we live accordingly, and have the powers of God-men," for it is precisely "in the degree that we open ourselves to this divine inflow are we changed from mere men into God-men."[42]

As we saw in chapter 2, the Yogi's powers, when taken seriously, fell into the rationalizing current of the meta-scientific concept of a universal energy. We have also seen that, from Mesmer's days onward, metaphysical practitioners have sought to use this energy toward therapeutic ends. Mind cure movements, as their label would suggest, tended to discard the material aspect of this energy altogether and instead advanced mind itself—which, given their Western ontologies, translated directly to spirit—as the all-pervading universal substratum of reality. In Yogananda's Indian metaphysical landscape, however, mind was by no means the final frontier. For this reason, though he found himself quite at home in New Thought and other mind cure circles, he nevertheless differentiated himself from these schools with quippy remarks, such as claiming that Yogoda did not amount to "thinking away disease, or mystic body or mind regulation" any more than it could be reduced down to "the science of physical culture as taught in gymnasiums and practiced in calesthenic clubs."[43] Indeed, Yogananda claims that Yogoda is unique among the various types of exercise science because it aims to focus attention not on physical aspects of muscle tension or bodily movements but on the flow of energy that underlies these somatic manifestations. His method entails a yoking of bodily movement, mental will, and spiritual energetic power to yield a system that "is the psycho-physiological clue, with a metaphysical touch, to the all-around growth of man."[44]

Yogoda is thus both distinct from and intimately related to the *haṭha* yogic practice of Kriya Yoga that belongs to Yogananda's lineage. Yogoda consists of Yogananda's calisthenic Energization Exercises followed by two more "advanced lessons" in concentration techniques that teach basic meditation by utilizing the Hong-Saw and Om *mantras*—the latter coupled with a simplified form of the *yoni mudrā*—that Yogananda adapted from Kriya Yoga practice. In this sense, Yogoda survives as the prerequisite to Kriya practice in the SRF's mail-order course. It is not surprising then that both systems ultimately rely on a similar logic of energy manipulation by way of psychosomatic cooperation via meditative focus. Furthermore, as we will shortly see, though Yogoda boasts many additional—and rather more practical—benefits, cosmic consciousness is not out of the question. However, the language through which practical and cosmic benefits are articulated is worlds apart, in no small way because it derives from two distinctly different discursive spheres.

Kriya Yoga, as it continues to be practiced by members of the SRF and as it was no doubt initially introduced to Yogananda's core group of devotees, retains a very recognizable *haṭha* yogic character. Energy—though there is no telling if Yogananda would have called it *prāṇa* or lifetrons—is channeled through the cakras by way of *prāṇāyāma* and *mantra* practice. The final goal is to concentrate this energy in the third eye in order to achieve oneness with the effulgent universal sound. In Yogoda, on the other hand, the practitioner awakens the energetic potential of his body by means of conscious muscular contraction and relaxation in order to hone his will. He thus creates a cooperative relationship between body, will, and mind through the conscious movement of nerve energy and is able to recharge his "body battery" from the infinite reservoir of the cosmos. Yogoda is advertised as a "tissue-will system of bodily perfection"[45] and no ecstatic states are explicitly mentioned. However, the ultimate goal of the concentration exercises is to put the practitioner "intuitionally in tune with the Cosmic Vibration."[46] How closely Yogananda understands such an attuned state to correspond to the traditional yogic state of *samādhi* is unclear.

What is clear from Yogananda's metaphysical adaptations of Indian practices is his reliance on the scientization of yogic superpower and the overall normalization of the superhuman Yogi. Because of Yogananda's devotional temperament, it is not unreasonable that he would have considered adherence to the ritual details of Kriya Yoga practice secondary to the effects of the practitioner's earnest and faithful intention. Considering his good-natured chastisement of Hamid Bey's glandular manipulation as a means to inducing trance states, we can safely deduce that Yogananda considered faith and devotion—or what he terms "love of God"—to be a far more powerful mechanism than those methods that relied entirely on technical expertise.

This would at first appear to be at odds with Yogananda's ongoing articulation of that his spiritual method was profoundly "scientific" in nature. Yogananda repeatedly claims that belief is only the initial necessary condition for "religion" and is therefore not at all synonymous with faith. One's religion is scientific insomuch as it is based on experimentation, and experimentation is above all practice. Faith requires practice, and practice requires will. Yogananda thus essentially updates Krishna's famous message to Arjuna in the *Bhagavad Gītā* when he declares that since one can never stop willing, one must hone one's will toward growth.

A New Yoga for the Willful Yogi

In Yogananda's words, Yogoda "combines the basic laws utilized by the ancient Hindu yogis, with the discoveries of modern physiological science."[47] As such, Yogoda—and consequently the Yogi whom it produces—is not only modern and scientific in its approach but also profoundly natural. Like Blavatsky and Vivekananda before him, Yogananda appeals to the ultimate unity of nature in order to render the supernatural as simply the logical extension of the natural. More than this, the supernatural is nothing but the natural in its truest form. Thus, Yogoda, relying on the basic laws of the universe—previously articulated in the occult wisdom of the ancient Yogis and rearticulated in the language of modern science in the West—caters to the natural potential of the human to become superhuman.

Yogananda's method is ultimately based on a seamless integration of auto-suggestive psychotherapy with physical calisthenics. He notes that "the yogis of India have a large number of postures which they practice in order to strengthen and develop their will,"[48] implicitly suggesting that his Energization Exercises are meant to accomplish the same goal as yogic *āsanas*. This is perhaps the clearest indication that we have from Yogananda as to his reasoning for not adopting the more commonly recognized forms of *āsanas*. It is likely that, as in the case of *khecarī mudrā* and the meditative posture *padmāsana*, he would have thought that *haṭha* yogic *āsanas*, which were associated in the Western mind with side-show contortions,[49] would be considered too bizarre or would simply be too difficult for his American students. What he retains, then, is not the form but the function of these "yogic postures," thus suggesting that there is a mutually beneficial relationship between the physical exercises that develop the power of will and the will itself, which in turn develops the capabilities of the body.

By 1923 the *Boston Post* was referring to Yogananda as "the Coué of gymnastics," implying that he had fully integrated the Yogoda system of Energization Exercises into his public demonstrations. Émile Coué (1857–1926), a French psychologist known for popularizing optimistic autosuggestion, rose to great popularity in Europe and subsequently in America, where he enjoyed the patronage of Anne Vanderbilt. However, Coué-style autosuggestion was only a single aspect of Yogananda's larger system. As he himself insisted:

> The famous Coué formula and theory are based on a partial understanding of the hidden factors behind many physical ailments. But the Coué formula cannot help many types of unimaginative minds, because it is based on the mistaken idea that imagination, rather than will, is the seat of many physical ills. In the last analysis, imagination is but a servant of the will.[50]

The above statement is ultimately a misreading of Coué insofar as it appears to misunderstand what Coué means by "imagination." However, the misunderstanding arises from Yogananda's much more expansive understanding of will. For Coué, the imagination, which he takes to mean something generally synonymous with the unconscious, and the will, which is simply the conscious resolve or desire, are oppositional forces. However, the imagination is exponentially more powerful than the will, and when the two are in conflict the "force of the imagination is in direct ratio to the square of the will."[51]

Yogananda disagrees, interpreting Coué's use of imagination perhaps a bit too literally and instead declaring will to be paramount.[52] This is primarily because he defines will not as "physical or mental strain or strenuousness" but as a "cool, calm, determined, increasingly steady and smooth flowing effort of the attention and the whole being toward oneness with a definite goal."[53] In other words, for Yogananda will begins to look a lot like meditative focus, thus betraying close kinship with Haddock's work. Even more than this, will writ large is "the essence of life" and "the determining factor of evolution."[54] It is "the initiator . . . the executor . . . the genius-maker" because "man cannot think without *willing to think*; far less can he act without *willing to act*. Will may be blind without intellect, but intellect is *powerless* and *worthless* without will."[55] This may all seem like a naïve oversimplification of conscious subjective agency until one considers Yogananda's claims in light of the metaphysical schema discussed in chapter 2. Will, for Yogananda, is directly instantiated in the electricity of nerve force. Consequently, it is energetically continuous with the very fabric of reality.

Nevertheless, it is significant that Yogananda lauds the Yogoda method as not only one that "enables you to see the VITAL FORCE, to hear the COSMIC VIBRATION, and thru a definite simple technique, to reach the Omnipresent Source of Infinite Power" but also one that "PUTS ON or TAKES OFF FAT, as desired, without trouble or delay."[56] In the spirit of what Singleton has aptly described as "an efficient merger of the cosmic and the cosmetic,"[57] Yogananda is ever attentive to note that that Yogoda has a range of distinctly physical benefits such as reviving the muscles, working to "strengthen injured or undeveloped osseous or bony structures," and teaching one how to "accelerate involuntary functions, such as those of the heart, the lungs, the stomach and intestines, the capillaries, the lymphatic glands, the veins, the cerebro-spinal axis (brain and spine), etc."[58] However, it accomplishes all of this by "spiritualizing the body by teaching one how to recharge the cells from inner cosmic energy." In the final analysis, the goal remains rather lofty in that through its "scientific technique of meditation (specific concentration applied to God) it leads to the bridging of the imaginary gulf existing between human and cosmic consciousness due to ignorance."[59]

By integrating physiological benefits and addressing the most mundane of concerns, Yogananda successfully insinuates his method into an increasingly secular and practically minded spiritual market. Bernard and his wife, Blanche De Vries, had already achieved popular acclaim for their coupling of yogic metaphysical principles with cosmetic goals, thereby establishing the corollary that a beautiful body was both a necessity for and a signal of an enlightened nature.[60] Yogananda did not fail to capitalize on this principle.

Later editions of the Yogoda pamphlets become increasingly lengthy and elaborate in their commercial claims. The ninth edition contains the following rather extensive list of ancillary "facts" about the technique:

1. It teaches how to recharge and release the body battery any time, at will.
2. No change of dress or place is required. Its basic principal exercises can be practiced without attracting attention—while on chair or sofa—lying, standing, sitting, or moving.
3. It can be most profitably applied to all forms of physical and concentration or meditation exercises.
4. It teaches how to improve (a) Beauty of form; (b) Grace of expression; (c) Centre of consciousness; (d) The power of mental receptivity.
5. It teaches how to prevent hardening of arteries and to insure lasting youth by stimulating an even circulation and helping eject foreign matter from the system.
6. It teaches how to quickly drive away headaches and how to harmonize all muscle actions.
7. It is an important accessory to art—improving voice (a help to musicians), steadying the nerves in violin playing, etc.
8. While waiting for the trolley car you will not catch cold, if you practice "Yogoda."
9. It teaches you how to exercise those parts which you think you cannot exercise.
10. IT TEACHES YOU HOW TO PUT ON OR TAKE OFF FAT.
11. It teaches you to make success out of failure, thru intelligent control of your own will forces.
12. It teaches you to control your material and spiritual destiny by tuning in with cosmic consciousness or the inexhaustible storehouse of cosmic supply.[61]

To the casual observer, Yogoda attempts to be a cure-all solution, guaranteed to transform one into a lithe, ever-youthful virtuoso in full control of both his body fat and his spiritual destiny. Having tapped into the interests and concerns of his target demographic, Yogananda pitches a modern form of holistic self-help aimed at professional urbanites, who might be just as occupied with catching cold while waiting for the trolley as they are with maximizing their cosmic potential. Moreover, Yogananda is clear in positioning his method in the context of physical culture, positively contrasting it with contemporary German techniques that require machinery and props. His claim regarding the practice's virtue of not attracting attention seems especially ironic, however, in light of the proliferation of anecdotes from his devotees detailing the occasions on which Yogananda embarrassed many a bystander and a few agents of the police. It was apparently a particular habit of his to launch into the Energization Exercises in the midst of public spaces.

Bridging Human and Superhuman

It is important to emphasize, however, that the promises of Yogananda's method also transcended simple cosmetics. His lectures touted "Scientific Control of Death, Disease—Everlasting Youth" and carried titles like "Mastering the Subconscious by Superconsciousness . . . Your Super Powers Revealed."[62] The demonstrations that accompanied these lectures—stopping and restarting the heart, hurling a group of men across the stage with a single muscle spasm—were clearly meant to illustrate the superhuman potential that lay at the heart of Yogoda practice.

Yogananda was profoundly invested in establishing the natural continuum between the ordinary human man (or woman) and the superhuman Yogi. Flyers for a series of lectures delivered at his Mt. Washington center in 1926 proclaimed the following subject matter:

Oct. 11: "Miracles of Yoga"
Its Western misconceptions. The powers and secrets of the Great Hindu Saints and Yogis given to you for your personal use and upliftment.

Oct. 13: "Christ, Christna, Buddha"
Your Divine Heritage! Every man can arouse the infinite forces of his being to achieve the high destiny of immortality! . . . How To Be Like Them in This Life. The practical application of their teachings to modern life. How to rise above pain and limitation and realize your true nature of omnipotence.

Oct. 14: "Quickening Human Evolution"
Luther Burbank has proved the natural evolution of plant life can be quickened by hundreds of years. Swami teaches that an intelligent cooperation with Cosmic Law can quickly regenerate mankind.

Oct. 15: "My Great Master"
A Living Son of God. His Life and Miraculous Powers as I saw them. He is still living in India and has attained to mastery over himself and the forces of nature.

Oct. 16: "Using Super Electrons for Your Highest Success"
Learn to Contact God in Every Activity and Detail of Your Life. Feel His
Presence as a Great All-Enveloping Mantle of Bliss, Energy and Thrilling
Life. . . . Greatest and Amazing Demonstration for Recharging Body
Battery.

Oct. 17: "Divine Healing by Holy Ghost Christ Power and Yogi Method"
Bring your sick friends. The Swami will intone chants invoking the presence of the Great Masters and Yogic Saints of the World, as Christ,
Christna, and Buddha. Thousands have been liberated and healed of
bodily and mental sickness and the soul-suffering of ignorance.

Oct 18 "Breaking the Bars of Fate by Soul-Force"
Control Your Destiny Thru the Infinite Powers Given You by the Creator!
Overcome Environment, Heredity, and Bad Habits Thru the Untapped
Source of Limitless Strength Within! Learn How to Solve Your Problems,
Spiritual, Matrimonial and Business.

Volumes could be written on Yogananda's creative spelling of Krishna as
"Christna" alone. Learning to bridge the gap between yoga, which Yogananda associated with Hindu traditions, and Christianity was instrumental to Yogananda's
mass appeal. This yielded the sustained use of eclectic terminology such as
"Christian Sat-Sanga" and "Yogoda Evangelism" in Yogananda's materials and is
evidenced in the meditations provided at the start of every issue of *East-West*, from
1932 onward, that read more like Christian prayers than any Indian style of meditation.[63] Given that Yogananda's headquarters were firmly situated in the spiritually
eclectic milieu of Los Angeles, birthplace of the Pentecostal Azusa Street Revival
only a few decades prior, it is possible that he was attempting to capitalize on lingering Evangelical fervor. The focus on "miraculous" healing forms a curious point
of intersection between American metaphysical and Evangelical spiritual currents.

However, in this context the use of Christianity also plays a larger purpose: to
establish the unity of religious goals as culminating in the state of perfected superhumanity. Likewise, the lectures, taken as a whole, demonstrate the breadth of
Yogananda's eclectic syncretism. In the course of a week's worth of lectures, we
discover that Jesus, Krishna, and the Buddha are all representatives of a single class
of "Great Masters and Yogic Saints," a class that every human being can join by
tapping into his or her "true nature of omnipotence" to "achieve the high destiny
of immortality" just as Yogananda's living teacher had done. Not only this, but the
entire enterprise is entirely scientific—akin to the mechanically accelerated evolution of plant life—and the average person is only steps away from being able to

use "Super Electrons" for everything from achieving the aforementioned immortality to solving his or her business and marital problems.

Yogananda's goal, like that of his predecessors, is to universalize the figure of the Yogi. In his *Autobiography*, he remarks:

> A swami, formally a monk by virtue of his connection with the ancient order, is not always a yogi. Anyone who practices a scientific technique of God-contact is a yogi; he may be either married or unmarried, either a worldly man or one of formal religious ties. A swami may conceivably follow only the path of dry reasoning, of cold renunciation; but a yogi engages himself in a definite, step-by-step procedure by which the body and mind are disciplined, and the soul liberated. Taking nothing for granted on emotional grounds, or by faith, a yogi practices a thoroughly tested series of exercises which were first mapped out by the early rishis. Yoga has produced, in every age of India, men who became truly free, truly Yogi-Christs.[64]

He further notes, "there are a number of great souls, living in American or European or other non-Hindu bodies today who, though they may never have heard the words yogi and swami, are yet true exemplars of those terms."[65] Building on the existing trope of the Theosophical Mahatmas, more commonly called simply "Great Masters" or "Perfected Masters" by the metaphysically minded individuals that circulated in Yogananda's company,[66] Yogananda declared that yogic attainment was universal, though the term itself might be particular. The use of the science of "yoga" then was simply to provide a more efficient means by accelerating a natural human inclination toward spiritual evolution.

Relying on this principle of universality and the primacy of intentional practice over tradition and formal ritual, Yogananda effectively takes up the "householder Yogi" motif that had been used by his predecessors and contemporaries from Vivekananda to Yogendra and had been embodied in his own lineage by Lahiri Mahasaya, and he invokes this motif as a marketing tactic for his target demographic of educated urban disciples. He goes so far as to actually redefine *rāja yoga* as follows:

> Yoga means uniting Mind-Power with Cosmic Power. Raja Yoga consists of those principles of concentration which were easily practiced even by the Rajas or royalists of India who were engrossed with the multifarious duties of their states.
>
> These methods of concentration, or Raja Yoga, which bring power over one's own destiny and which can turn failure—material, moral,

social or spiritual—into success can fit in with the busy and worried life of the American Rajas and Maharajahs, the American millionaires and billionaires.[67]

Elsewhere, Yogananda refers to yoga as "a middle path between complete renunciation and complete worldliness."[68] He must have realized that calls to renunciation would not go far amidst his American audiences, who were accustomed to New Thought rhetoric of material well-being as a sign of cosmic attunement. Instead, he agreed that health and wealth could very well be compatible with spiritual advancement if viewed in the correct light. Relying on a metaphysical version of the prosperity gospel, Yogananda taught that "business life need not be a material life. Business ambition can be spiritualized. Business is nothing but serving others materially in the best possible way."[69] Capitalistic productivity had to be balanced with a spiritual mindfulness.

It is exactly in this spirit that Yogananda, in an issue of *East-West*, lauded Henry Ford for inaugurating "a new era in spiritualizing business life by proposing a five day work week."[70] Given a two-day weekend, allowing for both leisure and spiritual development, the American businessman could effectively become a spiritual superman. The goal in short was to bridge the gap between the lofty promises of enlightenment and superpowers with the interests and exigencies of modern living. Neoliberal self-determination easily translated into metaphysical self-realization. Yogananda thus promised a spiritual practice that not only acknowledged the modern secular context of consumer capitalism but sought to maximize the individual's success within it. His vision, springing from the New Thought-inflected prosperity metaphysics of the Progressive Era, prefigured the spiritual consumerism of the New Age movement apart from which modern yoga culture cannot be understood.

From this perspective, Yogananda's *Autobiography* is a marked departure from the larger body of his work. Rather than dealing with the practical goals of stress management, weight loss, and even the subtler energetics of the Yogoda system, the *Autobiography* sets its sights much higher. It locates itself quite firmly in India, the land of Yogis, miraculous powers, and enlightenment. Its narrative understandably reflects a different trajectory of Yogananda's life than is revealed by other sources. However, it also offers a much more extensive elaboration of Yogananda's metaphysics than had previously been available in his earlier body of work discussed thus far in this study. In this sense, the *Autobiography* offers the second half of the equation representing Yogananda's reinterpretation of traditional yogic metaphysics just as it provides the second half of his life's narrative.

5

Hagiography of a Yogi

*I killed Yogananda long ago. No one dwells in this body now
but God.*

—PARAMAHANSA YOGANANDA

*Many autobiographies replete with famous names and color-
ful events are almost completely silent on any phase of inner
analysis or development. One lays down each of these books
with a certain dissatisfaction, as though saying: "Here is a
man who knew many notable persons, but who never knew
himself."*

—PARAMAHANSA YOGANANDA, *Autobiography of a Yogi*

THE TWO STATEMENTS above, both by Yogananda, reflect the central
paradox that characterizes his *Autobiography of a Yogi*. Despite the apparent
promise of its genre, the book actually contains relatively little information
about Yogananda himself. Indeed, the majority of the work is dedicated to
telling the stories of other men and women—other Yogis—whom Yogananda
found to be spiritually notable or didactically useful. At first glance, it might
seem like Yogananda has fallen into his own trap and filled his narrative with
"famous names and colorful events" at the cost of ignoring or willfully concealing his own inner life. And yet the title of the book is not *Autobiography of
Paramahansa Yogananda*. As I have argued, Yogananda saw himself first and
foremost as a Yogi. This reflects not only his conscious and subconscious shaping of his persona to adhere to the cultural archetype of the Yogi figure, as discussed in chapter 3, but also his broader belief that to be a Yogi was ultimately
to lose one's limited sense of ego-bound identity in absolute union with the
divine. Thus, Yogananda's identity as a Yogi is reflected not only in his own life
but in the lives and stories of other Yogis, for they are not in the final analysis
separate from his own.

Keeping this in mind, it is important to note exactly which parts of his own
life Yogananda chooses to discuss and which parts remain unmentioned. Gone

are the many associates who no doubt played pivotal roles in his progress both in India and abroad. Understandably there is no mention of the tempestuous rifts and legal struggles with Dhirananda and Nirad Ranjan Chowdhury. Nor is there any mention of the American Yogis who accompanied Yogananda on his lecture tours—not only the colorful Hamid Bey and Roman Ostoja but also the many core disciples who were instrumental to Yogananda's early success. These omissions are reflected in the simple logistics of the book's subdivisions: thirty-six of the eventual forty-nine chapters are concerned with events prior to Yogananda's arrival in America. Seven of the thirteen remaining chapters concern his return to India. Thus, in all, only six of the forty-nine chapters reflect Yogananda's life in the West—roughly 10 percent of the entire book. In reality, however, this time period accounts for nearly 50 percent of Yogananda's life. Approximately thirty of his fifty-nine years were spent on American soil.

Why, then, the apparent imbalance? It might be said that, for Yogananda as for his American audience, the Yogi together with his superpowers ultimately resides in the mystical distance of the Orient. This is perhaps partially true. And yet Yogananda's message is based primarily on the universality of yoga as an expression of human potential. Although his stories of saints and miracles are primarily staged in India, he makes it a point to dedicate entire chapters to the Catholic stigmatic Therese Neumann and the American Luther Burbank, the "Saint Amidst the Roses." There is, however, one very singular thing that exists for Yogananda only in India: his relationship with his guru.

There are many ways to read the *Autobiography*. One can glean quite a few endearingly prosaic observations from its pages. For instance, Yogananda's passion for food—substantiated by his disciples' accounts of his culinary talents and creative use of meat substitutes as well as the ubiquitous littering of recipes throughout the volumes of *East-West*—can be observed in the *Autobiography*'s detailed descriptions of every meal. One also notices a charming predilection for plant life, as witnessed by Yogananda's admiration for Jagadis Chandra Bose and Luther Burbank as well as the many smaller references that are no doubt artifacts of his aborted ventures into an agricultural education. These details are perhaps the closest that the *Autobiography* brings us to Mukunda Lal Ghosh, the man.

However, the book is self-professedly not about the man but about the Yogi. The *Autobiography* is not a novel, strictly speaking, but it does have a principal narrative arc. Its structure pivots on the relationship between Yogananda and his guru, Sri Yukteswar, as a reflection of the broader theme of Yogananda's spiritual progression. The chief "drama" of the work is to be found here. Tangential to this plot line, the *Autobiography* has two semi-didactic concerns: an exploration of the role of superpowers in relation to what it means to be a Yogi, and a metaphysical treatise.

In this sense, the text is also an auto-hagiography. Robin Rinehart coined this term to describe the writings of Rama Tirtha, a known and significant influence upon Yogananda, and the ways in which they reflect Rama Tirtha's hopes to "shape the way people would remember him"[1] and "chronicle reflexively his own experience of himself as a spiritually advanced person."[2] Timothy S. Dobe has expanded this notion to include auto-hagiography's reliance on "strategies of self-assertion that work through exemplarity and lineage" and thus constitute a "narrative practice that helps position the singular saint amid a host of better known holy men and women."[3] In Yogananda's case, this is all certainly true. His concern with lineage should be seen not only in terms of the authority it provides from both a traditional South Asian and a Western standpoint but also as reflecting a fundamental aspect of his identity. Yogananda consciously constructs a self-reflexive narrative of his self-discovery and spiritual growth in the ongoing tradition of powerful and spiritually enlightened Yogis ranging from the ancient ṛṣis to his guru and the other realized masters he encounters in the course of the narrative. The exploration of superpowers and their underlying metaphysics thus serves a related function by contextualizing the Yogi not just among his peers but also in the cosmos as a whole.

Finally, it should be noted that contrary to Dobe's statement above, many of Yogananda's accounts concern individuals that can hardly be considered "better known holy men and women." Some certainly are, as in the case of Gandhi or Neumann. Others, however, not only would have been unknown to the average American reader but are hardly represented as exemplary by Yogananda. Here one thinks of the Perfume Saint, whom we will meet shortly, or the random unnamed Yogi described to Yogananda by the police officer who interrupts his first flight from home. Since the fame of this Yogi, whose arm is mistakenly chopped off by the same police officer only to miraculously grow back three days later, never extends past a newspaper clipping presented to Yogananda, it is difficult to argue that he is meant to serve a real legitimating function. Rather, this story resembles the anecdotal asides that proliferate in travel narratives and memoirs of the period. The list of literature enumerated by Davis at the outset of chapter 3 of this study was of interest not only to spiritual seekers looking east for ancient wisdom but also to more casual audiences who were simply dazzled by the sights and wonders of the Orient. The crowning jewel of such literature, Brunton's *A Search in Secret India* (1934), which comprises a journalistic memoir of the author's encounters with Indian Yogis and wonder-workers, features precisely such narratives. The structure of Yogananda's book, especially with regard to the significant portions occupied with stories of Yogis and their superpowers, bears a striking similarity to Brunton's bestseller.

Satyeswarananda, one of Yogananda's more critical biographers, claims that as many as four American professional writers were charged with the job of editing the *Autobiography*. Yogananda himself acknowledges Laurie V. Pratt (Tara Mata) for her "editorial labors," as well as three other disciples who contributed materials, suggestions, and encouragement. This does not, of course, diminish the value of Yogananda's work—everyone needs an editor. As a result, however, Satyeswarananda observes:

> Now it seems that many additions, alterations, and changes were made in the process of writing the book. Ideas were interjected to look as if some divine hands were working behind the scenes. Mystifications were well thought out during the ten long years period of editing the forty-nine chapters from the materials Yogananda had collected. It was written with mystic vibrations which would be attractive to Christians.[4]

It is true that Yogananda's version of events does not always correspond with that of his other biographers. However, it seems that much of this could be attributed to perspective. For instance, while it may be objectively true that Sri Yukteswar was instructed to seek out Yogananda in Benares by concerned family members, such a fact need not nullify Yogananda's own sense of the cosmic significance of this meeting with the man who would become his guru. However, Satyeswarananda's point is well taken: it does indeed appear that the narrative is being guided by some greater force. Of course, in a sense, a narrative of any kind is by definition the imposition of a subjective order upon a series of otherwise random events. To narrativize something is to give meaning to raw experience. Some may even argue that there is no experience prior to narrative. Beyond this, Yogananda is very clear about his sense of a divine plan being worked out in his spiritual progress. He states this explicitly and repeatedly. Indeed, this premise lies at the very core of his work. Even so, as in all of his other writings, Yogananda was acutely aware of his audience, and his choice of language often reflects this awareness. His keen devotion to the maternal Kālī, for instance, becomes framed within an acknowledgment of the "Heavenly Father." Nevertheless, the *Autobiography* ultimately presents a coherent narrative of Yogananda's identity as a Yogi, in all of its cosmic and at times human significance.

Brief Note on the History of the Autobiography

As already mentioned, it can hardly be said that Yogananda's *Autobiography* was a solitary labor. In addition to including direct excerpts from Richard

Wright's travel diary, Yogananda himself acknowledges that he received much editorial assistance in producing the final published work. However, since Yogananda's death the *Autobiography* has undergone further revisions, which it is doubtful that Yogananda himself either made or approved. The book was first published in 1946 by The Philosophical Library and went through four editions before the rights to the text were acquired by the SRF in 1953. The third edition, released in 1951, includes several revisions, the most notable of which is an extra chapter that accounts for the final decade of Yogananda's life, aptly titled "The Years 1940–1951."[5] This may in fact be the definitive edition of the *Autobiography*. It is the most complete account published during Yogananda's lifetime and it is almost certain that he himself would have approved any changes made therein.

However, beginning with the fifth edition in 1954, several editorial changes have been made to the images and text of the book.[6] The SRF acquired the publishing rights to the *Autobiography* and has been responsible for the printing of the book since this time. Photos have been deleted, added, and modified (for example, Lahiri Mahasaya appears robed, whereas in prior editions he had appeared bare-chested). Most of the changes are minor and probably innocuous. Others, however, appear to be more ideologically charged. For instance, the initial editions mention that during the opening ceremonies at the Los Angeles Lake Shrine in 1951, "the audience then witnessed a remarkable demonstration of SRF boys of scientific asanas (postures) for health of body and mind."[7] However, this mention of postural practice is omitted from the text beginning with the sixth edition, and one cannot help but think that this may have much to do with the SRF's reluctance to acknowledge or propagate the postural element of Yogananda's lineage.[8] The seventh edition in 1956 brings a major overhaul with minor changes applied to nearly every page, nominally justifying most of these by citing edits that were made by Yogananda prior to his death but were not previously incorporated due to the expense of typesetting.

The most troubling changes include modified wording that seems to explicitly depart from Yogananda's original text. Mentions of Yogananda's goal to establish World-brotherhood Colonies are removed,[9] many mentions of the SRF are added, and the position and status of the householder Yogi is diminished.[10] At the same time, I was dismayed to find that one of my favorite quotes—"the law of miracles is operable by any man who has realized that the essence of creation is light"[11]—is nowhere to be found in the original editions. The changes are too numerous to effectively catalog here (especially when one takes into account the fact that some of the original edits have been edited numerous times since), and such a project is perhaps not directly relevant to the present study. Suffice it to say that the *Autobiography* has remained a living document that now, in its thirteenth edition, reflects the institutional position of the SRF as much as it does Yogananda's own account as far as the author's life and teachings are concerned.

Having discussed the biographical details of Yogananda's life as they appear outside of the *Autobiography* in chapter 3, I will not return to them here except briefly in addressing Yogananda's concern with yogic superpowers. Likewise, in discussing Yogananda's metaphysical framework, I will make some references to external sources, such as those covered in chapter 2, to establish context and illustrate the innovative nature of his synthesis. Otherwise, there is much to be gained from allowing Yogananda's narrative to speak for itself. Given the auto-biographical nature of the work, some consideration will necessarily be given to authorial intent, but the following analysis will remain largely structural in nature.

The Boy Who Wanted Superpowers, Revisited

All sources seem to confirm that Yogananda was a naturally spiritual child. It is unclear—and perhaps unlikely—that he ever pursued yogic superpowers strictly for their own sake. However, pursue them he did. This desire is never voiced explicitly in his own account, but the preponderance of episodic narratives fea-turing Yogis and their superhuman feats betray his fascination.

Satyeswarananda recounts the reaction of a devotee of the Ramakrishna Mission upon examining a Bengali translation of the *Autobiography*:

> I opened the title, *Yogikathamrit* and I could not continue to read it even a few pages. The book appeared to me as if it was a book of demonstration or application of *asta sidhai* [the eight classical yogic superpowers]. As I understand, the utilization and exhibition of *asta sidhai* are hindrances to realizing the Lord. At least, that is what I understand reading our sacred book *Sri Ramakrisna Kathamrit*.[12]

This is perhaps not an altogether inaccurate description of the book's contents. Almost half of Yogananda's *Autobiography* reads like a sort of travel narrative revolving around meetings with an array of superpowerful Yogis. However, the reader quickly discovers that not all supermen (or women) are created equal. At one extreme we have self-realized beings such as Sri Yukteswar, who rarely takes any credit for the phenomena he produces, preferring to attribute his healing abilities to divine will or the influence of astrological paraphernalia. At the other extreme reside unenlightened men like Afzal Khan, the fakir who was granted his powers as a blessing but went on to abuse them for petty thievery. Between the two poles rest some more ambiguous characters, such as Gandha Baba, or the "Perfume Saint."

The encounter with Gandha Baba is perhaps the best example of Yogananda's ultimate position on superhuman powers. The Perfume Saint appears to have had a very particular skill, consisting of the ability to produce any aroma at will, floral perfumes being his specialty. Yogananda initially suspects that Gandha Baba may have simply "induced an auto-suggestive state" or, in simpler terms, hypnotized him, until his sister is likewise able to perceive the smell of jasmine emanating from an otherwise scentless flower. However, Yogananda remains unconvinced of the utility of making flowers smell like other flowers. Gandha Baba is also able to materialize objects at will, an ability that Yogananda discovers anecdotally when a friend mentions having seen the Yogi materialize tangerines at a party. Although such displays have understandably made Gandha Baba quite popular, Yogananda concludes that "a guru too literally 'marvelous' was not to [his] liking"[13] and denounces "ostentatious displays of unusual powers."[14] He closes the account with a sentiment that echoes the traditional position also voiced by the Ramakrishna devotee quoted above: "Wonder-workings such as those shown by the 'Perfume Saint' are spectacular but spiritually useless. Having little purpose beyond entertainment, they are digressions from a serious search for God."[15]

The example of Gandha Baba is immediately followed by an account of the "Tiger Swami," or Sohong Swami, whose story demonstrates a somewhat different trajectory. The Tiger Swami stands as a perfect example of the intersection between yoga and physical culture that was only beginning to take root at this time. He gives voice to a concept that would come to form the core of Yogananda's teachings in America: the power of the mind to effect changes in the development of the body. The Tiger Swami explains:

> Mind is the wielder of muscles. The force of a hammer blow depends on the energy applied; the power expressed by a man's bodily instrument depends on his aggressive will and courage. The body is literally manufactured and sustained by mind.[16]

Having discovered this principle, the Tiger Swami proceeds to utilize his newfound mental powers and bodily strength in pursuit of fame and self-edification. As his name indicates, he had made his fortune by wrestling tigers until a particularly difficult match and a fateful illness turned him to the monastic path where he would thenceforth "subdue the beasts of ignorance roaming in jungles of the human mind."[17] Yogananda leaves impressed both by the Tiger Swami's earlier physical prowess and his subsequent spiritual turn. It appears that the initial materialism of the Tiger Swami's path, otherwise quite as ostentatious as that of the Perfume Saint, is redeemed by the ultimate realization that arises out of it.

Then there is the tale of Giri Bala, "The Woman Yogi Who Never Eats," which comes at the very end of Yogananda's narrative. Unlike Therese Neumann, who is likewise famous for her nonexistent diet, Giri Bala's condition stems from a rather quotidian source. Having grown up with an insatiable appetite, she was relentlessly shamed by her mother-in-law for her "gluttonous habits." One day Giri Bala could no longer abide the continuous reproaches and declared her resolution to never again touch food. The mother-in-law was understandably skeptical, and Giri Bala set off in a desperate search to discover the means to uphold her vow. Her prayers were answered when a Yogi master appeared and taught her a certain technique that would allow her to live without need of any food or water. Yogananda inquires why she has not taught others this method, to which Giri Bala replies that her guru instructed her to keep the technique forever secret so as not to interfere with the karmic drama of creation. To Yogananda's question of why she has thus been singled out to live without nourishment, she answers: "To prove that man is Spirit. . . . To demonstrate that by divine advancement he can gradually learn to live by the Eternal Light and not by food."[18] In this statement echoes the refrain of nearly every Yogi with whom Yogananda comes into contact— including even the theatrical Gandha Baba, who responds to Yogananda's jest that he will put the perfume companies out of business: "I will permit them to keep their trade! My own purpose is to demonstrate the power of God."[19] Time and again, the Yogis encountered by Yogananda assert that they exhibit their superpowers as testament to the power of the divine. Even Giri Bala's initially worldly motivation becomes transfigured into a manifestation of divine will.

It should be noted that the first two accounts—those of Gandha Baba and the Tiger Swami—are presented near the beginning of Yogananda's *Autobiography* and thus fall into his period of intensive spiritual exploration, whereas the third account of Giri Bala concerns an encounter that occurs upon his return to India approximately three decades later. It is clear that during this lengthy period his fascination with displays of superhuman power has remained unabated.

Stepping momentarily outside the present text, this sustained interest in superpowers and the accompanying explanations may go a long way toward illuminating Yogananda's predilection for including demonstrations of superhuman feats as highlights of his lectures in the West. Unlike Vivekananda, who firmly refused to succumb to the "put out or get out" attitudes of miracle-hungry audiences, Yogananda seemed only too eager to demonstrate the effects of his techniques of controlling and recharging the battery of the physical body. Although the line does begin to blur when considering his associations with the vaudeville circuit and stage magicians, perhaps Yogananda's theatrical flair can be attributed to his conviction that superhuman displays were sometimes necessary to instill faith in the doubting hearts of disciples. Tracing his spiritual journey as narrated in the *Autobiography*, it becomes abundantly clear that this method was instrumental in the solidification of his own convictions. If indeed anything changes in his attitude between the meetings with Gandha Baba and Giri Bala, it appears as a shift from skeptical wonder to weighed understanding.

Yogananda's own superhuman displays are, of course, never mentioned in the *Autobiography*, which goes no further than describing moments of divinely inspired intuition or miraculously answered prayers. It does not befit a Yogi to catalogue his own superpowers. However, Yogananda's education in becoming a proper Yogi is inextricably tied to the elaboration of his relationship with Sri Yukteswar. Interestingly, he does not fully surrender to Sri Yukteswar as his guru—despite claiming to recognize him as such upon their very first meeting—until Sri Yukteswar fulfills the condition to which he agreed upon accepting Yogananda as his disciple: to bestow upon him a vision of God, or *samādhi*. Restless, Yogananda seeks to once again escape to the Himalayas after only six months with Sri Yukteswar, admitting to ignoring his guru's "plain hint that he, and not a hill, was [his] teacher."[20] He finally returns, duly reprimanded by Ram Gopal Muzumdar, the "Sleepless Saint," who refuses to bestow *samādhi* upon him but intimates that his teacher will do so in due time. Yet even after the promised event solidifies Yogananda's commitment to his guru, the narrative proceeds to pivot on the continual interplay of doubt and reaffirmation between the two until the final climax of Sri Yukteswar's death and the resolution of his astral resurrection.

The Narrative Arc of a Spiritual Search

The very first sentence—and, more broadly, paragraph—of Yogananda's *Autobiography* is profoundly telling:

> The characteristic features of Indian culture have long been a search for ultimate verities and the concomitant disciple-guru relationship. My own path led me to a Christlike sage whose beautiful life was chiseled for the ages. He was one of the great masters who are India's sole remaining wealth. Emerging in every generation, they have bulwarked their land against the fate of Babylon and Egypt.[21]

Directly following this, he launches into vague recollections of a past life and memories of infancy and early childhood. Sri Yukteswar is not mentioned again for several chapters. The reader nevertheless knows from the very outset that Yogananda's search for truth will be indelibly tied to his search for this Christlike sage, whose identity remains hidden. The subsequent chapters are therefore filled with a sense of latent expectation. As we encounter the vast array of superpowerful Yogis, we must inevitably continue to ask along with Yogananda: "Is this my guru?"

The *Autobiography* is ruled, if not by a divine plan, then at least by a sense of long-spanning synchronicity. Yogananda's narrative works to highlight occurrences that might have otherwise appeared meaningless and to organize events that in themselves may be striking but gain even further import through mutual association. One of Yogananda's earliest memories is being miraculously healed of a near fatal case of Asiatic cholera by an image of his parents' guru, Lahiri Mahasaya. As the reader will soon discover, the legacy of Lahiri Mahasaya will continue to exert a significant, though initially subtle, influence on Yogananda's path. Despite his wide-ranging spiritual explorations, he ultimately finds himself situated within the same Kriya Yoga lineage into which his father first initiated him at the age of thirteen and which stems from the same guru whose image inexplicably saved his life at the age of eight.

There appear to be a number of events in Yogananda's earlier life that set him on the path of a spiritual seeker. He recounts four such experiences in the initial chapters of his work: the miraculous healing by means of Lahiri Mahasaya's image; a vision of the Himalayan Yogis and the divine effulgence of Īśvara, the Lord; his accidental magnification of his sister's boil, coinciding with the manifestation of a boil of his own; and the episode of the two kites obtained through devotion to the goddess Kālī. These experiences serve to illustrate Yogananda's realization of the power of the guru, the divine absolute, individual will, and devotion, respectively. However, although Yogananda is from an early age aware and desirous of powers that transcend the ordinary, his ambition to become a Yogi does not appear to fully manifest until the death of his mother.

Yogananda's mother passes away suddenly and unexpectedly when he is only eleven. Her death is an irreparable loss to the entire family but is especially devastating to the young Yogananda. However, with the death of his mother and thereby of his strongest earthly love comes a revelation of destiny. Yogananda is overcome by an intense longing, which becomes channeled into a restless spiritual ardor. He must go to the Himalayas. The mountains, representative of the Yogis who reside therein, become a lifelong beacon. Yogananda demonstrates his resolve with the first of many failed attempts to flee to the legendary site, but he is quickly retrieved by his eldest brother. However, even as his "heart wept for the lost Mothers, human and divine,"[22] his brother reveals to him a message that further galvanizes his conviction to become a Yogi. On her deathbed, his mother had delivered a revelation, to be passed on to Yogananda a year after her death. When Yogananda was still an infant, she took him to see the great Lahiri Mahasaya, who told her, "Little mother, thy son will be a yogi. As a spiritual engine, he will carry many souls to God's kingdom."[23] This destiny was subsequently confirmed to her by another *sādhu* who came to her shortly before her death, foretelling the event. It was also confirmed by the miraculous materialization of a silver amulet, which his mother was charged with delivering to Yogananda after her death by way of her eldest son. Upon receiving the object, Yogananda recounts:

> A blaze of illumination came over me with possession of the amulet; many dormant memories awakened. The talisman, round and anciently quaint, was covered with Sanskrit characters. I understood that it came from teachers of past lives, who were invisibly guiding my steps. A further significance there was, indeed; but one does not reveal fully the heart of an amulet.[24]

The amulet thus kindles within Yogananda the profound sense of destiny that would guide many of his pursuits. He refers in the first pages of the *Autobiography* to the lucid recollections "of a distant life, a yogi amidst the Himalayan snows"[25] that constituted his earliest memories in infancy. One can assume that the "distant memories" awakened by the amulet may have been of a similar nature. The amulet places Yogananda's quest within the framework of a larger spiritual journey, spanning multiple lifetimes and perhaps guided by multiple superhuman hands of gurus past and present.

After this revelation, Yogananda embarks on a wide-ranging spiritual search. It will be another five years until he finally finds his long-awaited guru in Sri Yukteswar. His tantric explorations, chronicled elsewhere, are alluded to in the following statement, illustrating the single-pointed nature of his ambitions:

> My promise to Father had been that I would complete my high school studies. I cannot pretend to diligence. The passing months found me less frequently in the classroom than in secluded spots along the Calcutta bathing ghats. The adjoining crematory grounds, especially gruesome at night, are considered highly attractive by the yogi. He who would find the Deathless Essence must not be dismayed by a few unadorned skulls. Human inadequacy becomes clear in the gloomy abode of miscellaneous bones. My midnight vigils were thus of a different nature from the scholar's.[26]

Although we know that his childhood friend, the future Swami Satyananda, occasionally accompanied him on these midnight excursions, this must have been a largely solitary practice for Yogananda. Like his attic meditation room, the Calcutta charnal grounds were host to young Yogananda's experiments with a personal *sādhana* that occasionally reached beyond the limits of social sanctions. However, not all of his efforts were similarly self-guided. During these years, Yogananda also sought out a number of well-known Yogis—whether as part of his search of a spiritual guru, or to satisfy a curiosity with superhuman powers, or most likely a good measure of both. The chapters that separate the death of his mother from his first meeting with Sri Yukteswar are among the most colorful— and for this reason the most popular—of the book, cataloguing a diverse roster of Yogis and their various talents.

Having miraculously obtained his high school diploma, Yogananda eventually resolves to leave home to devote himself fully to his search. However, he quickly finds himself alienated by the service-driven life of the Benares ashram to which he escapes. As his relationship with his fellow inmates continues to degenerate, he discovers that the silver amulet bequeathed to him by his mother has disappeared, as it was foretold to do once its purpose had been accomplished. Thoroughly despondent, Yogananda locks himself in the attic to sob and pray until some answer is granted. After several hours, a divine female voice informs him that his guru is to arrive this very day, so when a young monk calls him down to accompany him on an errand, Yogananda obediently ventures out. His hopes are finally fulfilled at the marketplace, where he spots a Swami who inspires in him a wave of preternatural recognition. Unsure, Yogananda walks on only to feel himself magnetically drawn back to the stranger as his feet literally begin to disobey him. They recognize each other immediately: "Gurudeva!" Yogananda exclaims—"O my own, you have come to me!" returns Sri Yukteswar.[27]

Yogananda's search appears to have found its consummation. Guru and disciple exchange vows of unconditional love. Then, to Yogananda's dismay, Sri Yukteswar instructs him to return home to Calcutta and declares that he will see Yogananda again in four weeks at his ashram in Serampore. As quickly as it was bestowed, the guru's affection is seemingly withdrawn as he tells Yogananda:

> Now I have told my eternal affection, and have shown my happiness at finding you—that is why you disregard my request. The next time we meet, you will have to reawaken my interest: I won't accept you as a disciple easily. There must be complete surrender by obedience to my strict training.[28]

Obstinate, Yogananda ignores Sri Yukteswar's instructions to return to Calcutta and instead returns to his residence to suffer three more weeks of hostility from the residents of the ashram. He finally resolves to leave, paying a visit to his eldest brother and the Taj Mahal in Agra and taking a short detour to Vrindavan, before finally arriving at Sri Yukteswar's ashram in Serampore exactly four weeks after their first meeting.

The second meeting, however, proves to be somewhat less harmonious than the first. Guru and disciple wrangle for over an hour regarding their mutual obligations to one another. Finally, Yogananda agrees to wholeheartedly accept Sri Yukteswar's authority in every detail of his life—which at this time largely involves his moving back to Calcutta and attending university—on the condition that his master will promise to reveal God to him.

Yogananda's descriptions of his time with Sri Yukteswar oscillate between retrospective exaltations and more chronologically situated accounts that belie a certain skepticism. Praise of the guru's appearance, wisdom, demeanor, and general character is interspersed with tales of the time he pinched Sri Yukteswar's nose during a nocturnal *samādhi* for fear that the older man had gone into cardiac arrest.

Yogananda's first conflict with Sri Yukteswar emerges six months into the discipleship, when the former requests to depart for the Himalayas, hoping "in unbroken solitude to achieve continuous divine communion."[29] When Sri Yukteswar calmly intimates that there are plenty of unenlightened "hill men" living in the Himalayas and that a geological formation is a poor substitute for a "man of realization" where wisdom is concerned, Yogananda simply repeats his query and, willfully misinterpreting his guru's silence for consent, takes off the following day. Like all of Yogananda's attempted flights from home, the excursion proves short-lived, arduous, and ultimately fruitless. He is quickly turned back by the other disciple of Lahiri Mahasaya from whom he had hoped to receive guidance and returns, humbled, to Sri Yukteswar.

To read Yogananda's relationship with Sri Yukteswar is to glimpse his perpetually unfulfilled longing. The feeling of something lacking—of not enough—is ever present in the subtext even as the narrative itself is delivered from the vantage point of an attained state of realization. Yogananda describes his meeting with Sri Yukteswar as a moment of cosmic consummation, yet six months later he is ready to abandon the relationship for a solitary search in the Himalayas. Upon his return, Sri Yukteswar bestows upon him a glimpse of cosmic consciousness by inducing a state of *samādhi*, yet a few months later Yogananda inquires when he will finally find God, not believing his guru's assertion that his search is already complete. On this point, Sri Yukteswar appears to offer a mild chastisement:

I am sure you aren't expecting a venerable Personage, adorning a throne in some antiseptic corner of the cosmos! I see, however, that you are imagining that the possession of miraculous powers is knowledge of God. One might have the whole universe, and find the Lord elusive still! Spiritual advancement is not measured by one's outward powers, but only by the depth of his bliss in meditation.[30]

The reference to powers is somewhat unexpected, given the tenor of Yogananda's descriptions of his spiritual search. The narrative never goes so far as to reference Yogananda's own desire for powers, though it is pointedly full of marvelous accounts of powers displayed by others, including Sri Yukteswar. Sri Yukteswar's response here is a possible hint that suggests Yogananda's dissatisfaction with his inability to manifest powers comparable to those of his guru, despite his success in achieving states of ecstatic meditation.

As for Yogananda's move westward, we are led to believe that Sri Yukteswar foresaw and blessed the decision as being in accordance with Yoganada's destiny. Indeed, Yogananda attributes the seeds of this idea to his guru's prescient hints rather than to any ambition of his own. Critics might say that in America Yogananda lost his way. Evidence of scandal is tantalizing and at times compelling but ultimately circumstantial. We learn little of his time on American soil if the *Autobiography* is taken as exclusive source material. Accounts appearing in *East-West* are more illuminating, though we can only guess as to the real reasons why Yogananda chose to largely exclude the details of a full three decades of his life from the final narrative of his journey. Yogananda's version of his brief return to India also belies external accounts of conflict. However, even in Yogananda's words, his homecoming to India is at best bittersweet.

Interestingly, Yogananda chooses not to describe the reunion with his guru through his own eyes and prose but excerpts instead from the travel diary kept by his disciple and ad hoc secretary on the trip, Richard Wright. Wright's account gives no hint of any trouble but catalogues a warm and heartfelt reception by both parties:

> No words passed in the beginning, but the most intense feeling was expressed in the mute phrases of the soul. How their eyes sparkled and were fired with the warmth of renewed soul-union! A tender vibration surged through the quiet patio, and even the sun eluded the clouds to add a sudden blaze of glory.[31]

In Yogananda's account of his final days with Sri Yukteswar, the longing once again becomes palpable. However, it is no longer a longing for power or greater enlightenment, but rather a very human desire for approval from his teacher. Upon Yogananda's return, there are no further accounts of spiritual lessons from his guru. Instead, Yogananda chooses to recount the morning on which he approached Sri Yukteswar with the following query:

> Guruji, I came to you as a high-school youth; now I am a grown man, even with a gray hair or two. Though you have showered me with silent

affection from the first hour to this, do you realize that once only, on the day of meeting, have you ever said, "I love you"?[32]

When Sri Yukteswar, albeit after some initial reluctance, declares to Yogananda his love for a student who has been nothing less than a son, Yogananda confides:

> I felt a weight lift from my heart, dissolved forever at his words. Often had I wondered at his silence. Realizing that he was unemotional and self-contained, yet sometimes I feared I had been unsuccessful in fully satisfying him. His was a strange nature, never utterly to be known; a nature deep and still, unfathomable to the outer world, whose values he had long transcended.[33]

The passage perhaps tempts a psychoanalytical interpretation, but such a reading would oversimplify the import of Yogananda's feelings toward Sri Yukteswar. Yogananda's relationship with his actual father comes across as rather more straightforward. After the tragic and early loss of his mother, Yogananda remarks that his father's affectionate nature blossomed and the man effectively fulfilled the roles of both parents. No love was thenceforth withheld. Yogananda's need for Sri Yukteswar's approval, however, is colored not only by the familial affection shared by the two men but also by Sri Yukteswar's spiritual authority and gravitas. Although Yogananda never states it outright, one imagines that his return to his guru after a full fifteen years must have brought along with it no small amount of anxiety. Even discounting the possibility that Yogananda may have had any doubts or regrets concerning his actions while abroad, he must surely have felt the weight of his mission before the eyes of his teacher. In another sense, this revelation of emotional anxiety serves to foreshadow the even greater uncertainty to come.

When only a few days later Sri Yukteswar divulges to Yogananda that his work on earth is coming to a close and that it is up to Yogananda to carry on, the latter responds with fear and subsequent denial. Despite Sri Yukteswar's fairly explicit statements, Yogananda observes only his robust appearance, stating: "Basking day by day in the sunshine of my guru's love, unspoken but keenly felt, I banished from my conscious mind the various hints he had given of his approaching passing."[34] Even as arrangements are made for the survival of Sri Yukteswar's estate and ashram, Yogananda begs him not to suggest that time may be in short supply. Suddenly he is struck with the conviction to attend the approaching Kumbha Mela in the hope of meeting the immortal Babaji. Willfully ignoring Sri Yukteswar's reluctance to have him depart, even when he plainly states that Babaji is unlikely to appear at the festival, Yogananda chooses to chase after a meeting with an immortal guru rather than witness the passing of a mortal one. Retrospectively, Yogananda writes:

> Apparently I was remaining oblivious to implications in Sri Yukteswar's attitude because the Lord wished to spare me the experience of being forced, helplessly, to witness my guru's passing. It has always happened in my life that, at the death of those dearly beloved by me, God has compassionately arranged that I be distant from the scene.[35]

In a footnote Yogananda indicates that he had likewise been absent for the death of his mother, eldest brother, eldest sister, father, and several close disciples. Of course Yogananda's distance during these times was hardly an accident. Whether ordained by a divine plan or not, most if not all of these absences—save the first during his mother's passing—can be attributed to his single-minded pursuit of his career as a Yogi.

Yogananda's narrative of his guru's passing is characterized by a continuous tug of war between retrospective prescience and immediate denial and disbelief. Having returned to Calcutta, he receives an urgent telegram telling him to rush to Serampore, where Sri Yukteswar has departed. Yet he insists that a divine internal voice instructs him not to depart that very night, as his prayers for his master's life cannot be granted, causing him not to board the train until the following evening. On the train he has a foreboding vision of a gravely visaged Sri Yukteswar, who only nods in response to his beseeching "Is it all over?" and silently disappears.[36] Arriving at the station, he still refuses to acknowledge the truth when a stranger approaches him to inform him of Sri Yukteswar's passing. The remainder of the chapter catalogues the subsequent events with an air of utter gloom. No amount of surety that Sri Yukteswar has departed at last into the bliss of cosmic consciousness is able to slake Yogananda's grief at the loss of his teacher. His passage back to America is cancelled due to insufficient space to accommodate the company's beloved Ford automobile, and he returns to Puri to mourn.

Sri Yukteswar's death is thus colored by Yogananda's denial and subsequent guilt. In light of their separation during the guru's final days, Yogananda's anxiety regarding Sri Yukteswar's love and approval becomes all the more urgent. The final vision of Sri Yukteswar received by him on the train to Serampore betrays this angst in its focus on the departed man's stern, perhaps even cold, countenance. The promise of divine union seems irrelevant and so lies forgotten.

Yogananda's despondency receives its first spark of relief about three months later, when Krishna suddenly appears to him on a rooftop across from the Bombay Regent Hotel. Although unable to decipher Krishna's message, Yogananda cites this as presaging some uplifting spiritual event. A week later, in the same hotel room, Sri Yukteswar manifests himself before the awestruck Yogananda in his astrally resurrected form. Immediately enveloping his guru in an "octopus grip," Yogananda exclaims: "Master mine, beloved of my heart, why did you leave me? . . . Why did you let me go to the Kumbha Mela? How bitterly have I blamed myself for leaving you!"[37] Instead of his earlier stern expression, Sri Yukteswar's face now wears an "angel-bewitching smile." He addresses Yogananda lovingly as his son. At last the reconciliation of Yogananda's guilt-driven anxiety is found, and with it arrives perhaps the most explicit revelation of metaphysical realization the book has to offer.

Sri Yukteswar's cosmological exposition is not entirely new. We have already been made privy to the basic elements of Yogananda's light-based metaphysics in previous chapters and have also been introduced to the idea of astral yogic resurrection (Lahiri Mahasaya) and immortality (Babaji). However, the placement of this uniquely lengthy metaphysical treatise is not unintentional. At this point, more than any other in the work, Yogananda's personal narrative works in perfect tandem with his didactic intent. We perceive the revelation of the work's cosmological schema through Yogananda's wonder-filled eyes as Sri Yukteswar describes his new state of being. Thus, the chapter effectively plays on the convergence of Yogananda's emotional attachment to his guru and his quest for spiritual knowledge and realization. The reader is compelled to accept the metaphysical exposition because, like Yogananda, she is both hungry for spiritual truth and has grown to trust and admire the figure who serves as its mouthpiece.

The Metaphysical Treatise

In addition to its narrative and biographical elements, the *Autobiography* also provides the fullest expression of Yogananda's metaphysical schema. Hints of this framework appear in *East-West* as well as in his other minor publications, but it is not until his master work that Yogananda provides us with a full exposition of the philosophical and metaphysical underpinnings of his worldview.

This schema, though referenced throughout the book, is developed in stages beginning with the chapter entitled "The Science of Kriya Yoga." There Yogananda explains the method of practice belonging to his tradition as an accelerated path of human evolution. In doing so, he links the practice to the authority of a scientific approach (as the title of the chapter suggests) while simultaneously introducing a metaphysical framework in which the evolution of the body is linked to a transformation on the astral, or subtle, level. This system is further developed a few chapters later in "The Law of Miracles," where Yogananda turns to popular scientific theory—specifically, an interpretation of Einstein's work and other contemporary concepts of electrodynamics—to provide a grounding for the subtle laws of nature that govern yogic practice and the resulting superpowers. This metaphysical exposition reaches its crescendo as a full-blown revelation delivered by the astrally resurrected Sri Yukteswar. Thus, the resolution of the narrative's primary "conflict"—that is, the vacillating relationship between Yogananda and his guru—corresponds to the resolution of the mystery that surrounds the physical possibility of the narrative's many wondrous occurrences. Yukteswar's resurrection serves not only as a final affirmation of the unbroken commitment between guru and disciple but also as an irrefutable testament to the reality of the metaphysical concepts the reader is finally made to understand.

In providing us with a full cosmology, Yogananda draws out a roadmap for the gradual perfection of the Yogi. In doing so, he introduces a typology of divinized or perfected beings. His overall schema proposes three types of bodies: (1) the idea or causal body; (2) the subtle astral body; and (3) the gross physical body. The latter includes self-realized human yogis whose bodies may show signs of perfection and who exhibit superhuman abilities in accordance with their degree of accomplishment. There are also, however, beings who inhabit astral bodies composed of *prāṇa* or, as Yogananda translates it, "lifetrons." These include "resurrected" bodies, which Yogananda treats as perfected forms willfully reconstituted from subtle elements but which may appear as gross matter. Still higher are causalbodied beings that exist beyond the "finer-than-atomic energies" of lifetrons[38] in "the minutest particles of God-thought."[39] Finally, there are beings who appear to be a conflation of traditional concepts of *siddha* and *avatāra*, existing outside of the aforementioned system of embodiment but choosing to manifest themselves and become embodied for a specific purpose.

Yogananda's tripartite system of embodiment appears to be closely modeled on a generic Vedāntin framework, which likewise consists of three aspects referred to as *kāraṇa śarīra* (causal body), *sūkṣma* or *liṅga śarīra* (subtle body), and *sthūla śarīra* (gross body). The two lower aspects are grounded in a basically Sāṃkhyan framework, with the gross body consisting of the *mahābhūtas*, or gross elements, and the subtle body encompassing the higher evolutes of *prakṛti* (everything from the *tanmātras*, the subtle elements, to the *buddhi*, intellect) in addition to three components—*kāma* (desire), *karma* (action), and *avidyā* (ignorance)—that reflect the binding aspects of subjectivity, along with five *prāṇas* (vital breaths).

Yogananda's system likewise includes a causal body, which he states is composed of the thirty-five ideas that result in the manifestations of the components of the two lower bodies. The first of these is the astral body, a term that he may have adopted from Theosophy or more likely from a more diffuse Western metaphysical context, which for him becomes synonymous with the subtle body as a whole.[40] This subtle body includes the typical aspects of intellect (*buddhi*), ego (*ahaṃkāra*), and mind (*manas*), to which Yogananda adds feeling. Below this are the five instruments of knowledge (*jñānendriyas*), five instruments of action (*karmendriyas*), and five instruments of lifeforce (most likely the *prāṇas*). The five subtle elements (*tanmātras*) are excluded. The gross body, in turn, consists not of the five gross elements (*mahābhūtas*) but of sixteen metallic and nonmetallic, or chemical, elements. It seems safe to assume that by these Yogananda means existing elements drawn from the standard periodic table, although no apparent explanation is given for their being sixteen in number.[41]

Yogananda introduces this system primarily to explain the various modes of embodiment available to the ascending levels of perfected beings. Even the gross physical body does not exclude a certain level of perfection. Throughout his narrative, Yogananda introduces the reader to a number of ordinary embodied Yogis who are nevertheless in possession of some fairly extraordinary superpowers. For instance, the body of Lahiri Mahasaya is said to exhibit superhuman features such as breathlessness, sleeplessness, and the cessation of the heartbeat even in his gross embodied state, and we meet a number of Yogis who are capable of multiplying their bodies to simultaneously appear in at least two locations prior to formally leaving their gross incarnations. Similarly, following his death and one day after his subsequent cremation, Lahiri Mahasaya, the "resurrected master, in a real but transfigured body" [42] is reported as appearing to three disciples in three different cities. The distinction between this body and the multiplied bodies of still-living Yogis is not made clear. However, we are told in no uncertain terms by both Lahiri Mahasaya and Sri Yukteswar that the resurrected body of the Yogi is a subtle astral body.

Astral bodies normally inhabit the astral universe, which is made up of many astral planets and is in fact hundreds of times larger than the physical universe. Yogananda compares the two to a hot air balloon, where the physical universe is the solid basket beneath the much larger, lighter, and more vibrant balloon of the astral universe. The causal universe in turn is not a manifest entity but the ideas of the other two universes, just as the causal body is composed of the thirty-five ideas that are reified into the elements of the astral and physical bodies. The astral universe is inhabited by all types of subtle beings, such as fairies, mermaids, fishes, animals, goblins, gnomes, demigods, and spirits, who all reside in different astral planes or planets "in accordance to their karmic qualifications."[43] Yogananda even describes an adapted picture of the long-standing Vedic conflict between the *devas* (gods) and the *asuras* (who are here called "fallen dark angels") as they wage constant war against each other with "lifetronic bombs or mental *mantric* vibratory rays."[44] On the whole Yogananda adapts and elaborates on the basic Swedenborgian model of multiple celestial realms that had already become popularized in America through iterations of the Spiritualist and Theosophical traditions.[45] However, he lends to it inflections that are both traditionally Indian and modern scientific in nature.

This entire exposition concerning the astral universe is delivered through the mouth of Sri Yukteswar, who informs Yogananda that he has been resurrected— not reincarnated but resurrected—on Hiranyaloka, which Yogananda translates as "Illumined Astral Planet."[46] This "subtler heaven" of Hiranyaloka is differenti- ated from the astral world at large in that it is a higher astral planet inhabited by highly spiritually developed beings who have mastered the meditative ability to consciously leave their physical bodies at death during their last incarnation. In other words, they have passed into the state of *nirvikalpa samādhi*, or uninter- rupted meditative absorption without physical awareness, while on earth. They have also passed through the ordinary astral spheres to which all earthly beings must go after death, where they have destroyed all of their binding *karma*— something that ordinary people cannot do because they are too entranced by the astral worlds to see any reason to engage in spiritual advancement.[47]

Yogananda's narrative gives us two examples of such advanced beings: Lahiri Mahasaya and Sri Yukteswar. It is important to note that both, when they reap- pear after their respective physical deaths, are described as "resurrected." When Lahiri Mahasaya appears to his disciple Keshabananda he states:

> From the disintegrated atoms of my cremated body, I have resurrected a remodeled form. My householder work in the world is done, but I do not leave the earth entirely. Henceforth I shall spend some time with Babaji in the Himalayas, and with Babaji in the cosmos.[48]

Likewise, when Yogananda asks the astral Sri Yukteswar whether his body, which seems tangible enough when Yogananda embraces him and even smells the same, is exactly like the body that had been buried only a short time ago, Sri Yukteswar replies:

> Yes, my child, I am the same. This is a flesh and blood body. Though I see it as ethereal, to your sight it is physical. From cosmic atoms I created an entirely new body, exactly like that cosmic dream physical body which you laid beneath the dream sands at Puri in your dream world. I am in truth resurrected—not on earth but on an astral planet.[49]

The astral body, although it is etheric or—as it is more commonly described by Yogananda, lifetronic—looks and feels as though it were physical when it appears in the physical world. Both Lahiri Mahasaya's and Sri Yukteswar's resur- rected bodies are described as "flesh and blood." However, the astral body is also described, like the *haṭha* yogic subtle body, as having an "astral brain," which is in reality a "thousand-petalled lotus of light," in addition to six awakened centers along the astral cerebro-spinal axis of the *suṣumnā*. Astral beings can materialize and dematerialize at will and assume any form they desire, at least for a time. In most cases, however, one's astral form is the exact counterpart of one's last physical form at the height of its youth, though on this point the astral Sri Yukteswar conveniently specifies that occasionally some choose to retain their aged appearance. Astral beings also possess a third astral eye, placed vertically on the forehead, which governs the sixth sense of intuition. By virtue of this sixth organ, astral beings can experience any sensation through any sense organ, resulting in a kind of synesthetic perception of reality.

Interestingly, this sixth organ, along with its corresponding sense capacity of intuition, appears nowhere in Yogananda's schema of the astral body, which tends to follow Sāṃkhyan notions of the traditional five sense organs fairly precisely. However, it may also be significant in this context that Yogananda's framework entirely excludes the five subtle elements (*tanmātras*). As previously noted, in Yogananda's work we see an interesting move toward a kind of quantum monism. Again and again, the text affirms that everything in the physical, astral, and even causal worlds is ultimately composed of light. On the astral level, this light congeals into the somewhat grosser particles of lifetrons, or *prāṇa*. This metaphysical move thus eliminates the need for a fivefold division of subtle elements, which now appear just as antiquated as the five gross elements from a molecular standpoint. However, given such a system, Yogananda's enumertion of the five traditional sense organs as well as the five organs of action appears rather out of place. After all, astral beings hardly rely on their traditional sense organs but instead employ the aforementioned sixth sense of intuition. Although Yogananda pays lip service to traditional Sāṃkhyan and Vedāntin categories in his metaphysical taxonomy, his more qualitative descriptions imply a much more Western metaphysical perspective, no doubt acquired during his sojourn among the New Thought and other metaphysically inclined circles in the United States.

A final aspect of Yogananda's treatment of the astral body relates to his reinterpretation of the idea of resurrection, which quite clearly derives from Christian influences and the Christian orientation of his intended audience. Yogi Ramacharaka, or Atkinson, had already described in his *Mystic Christianity* (1908) Jesus's resurrection as "the appearance in the Astral Body—the return from the Astral Plane in which He had sojourned for the three days following the crucifixion."[50] Likewise, in Yogananda's system resurrection is a function reserved for those who have consciously advanced to the astral world. Whereas reincarnation is the fate at death of all unenlightened beings, who enjoy a temporary and involuntary sojourn on the astral plane before their earthly *karma* draws them back into physical rebirth, those who have achieved the state of *nirvikalpa samādhi* in their final physical incarnation permanently advance to one of the astral planets in full consciousness of their trajectory. The physical body of the last incarnation is in this case "resurrected" as an astral body of lifetrons. Thus, Yogananda effectively combines Indian notions of the perfected body that a realized tantric *sādhaka* achieves by virtue of his practice and Christian notions of the resurrection body as a youthful and the perfected form of one's earthly self that is accessible at endtimes, as witnessed by the resurrected body of Jesus.

Yogananda's exposition about the causal body is comparatively much more brief. The causal body, which is made up of the minutest particles of differentiated God-thought, does not appear to have a visible form beyond that of pure light. Although causal bodies are still held together by desire, their desires are for perceptions only and are immediately satisfied due to their ability to spontaneously manifest anything through sheer thought. As there is no further differentiated schema to lay out, the astral Sri Yukteswar simply paints an impressionistic picture of causal-bodied beings whose "bright thought-bodies zoom past trillions of Spirit-created planets, fresh bubbles of universes, wisdom-stars, spectral dreams of golden nebulae on the skyey bosom of Infinity"[51] for as long as they choose not to or are unable to relinquish the final bonds of desire that delimit their subjectivities from the undifferentiated cosmic absolute.

Beyond Metaphysics

Up to this point, even at the level of the extremely subtle causal materiality, Yogananda has been dealing with the material world. Beyond this system of the three bodies (and their correlating universes), however, Yogananda also adopts a twofold classification of liberated beings: *jīvanmukta*, or "freed while living," and *paramukta*, or "supremely free."[52] The first term is never fully elucidated by Yogananda, but it seems safe to assume that this is the level of attainment that he wishes to ascribe to realized Yogis such as Lahiri Mahasaya and Sri Yukteswar. *Jīvanmukta*s enjoy the state of liberation while living for a limited time in their physical bodies, after which they cast off their mortal forms at the time of death and ascend to the higher astral realms. At the stage of *paramukta*, however, we find a superhuman conflation of *siddha* and *avatāra* that describes the one being who mostly closely approximates divine status in Yogananda's work: Babaji. The *paramukta* is a being who has completely surpassed the realms of *māyā* and rebirth—that is, he exists entirely beyond all three forms of embodiment. If the *paramukta* chooses to return to a human-like material body—which is, in accordance with the traditional notion of an *avatāra*, a rare occurrence having a very specific purpose—his body appears as a "light image" composed of lifetronic particles and not subject to *karma* or indeed any form of "universal economy."[53] This liberated body casts no shadow and leaves no footprint. In contrast to traditional Indian notions of *avatāra*, however, Yogananda's "avatar" is not simply a descent of the divine but a sort of "return" of a fully divinized individual self that nevertheless started out as fully human. According to Yogananda, Babaji's original patronymic and place of origin is not known.[54] Babaji can, of course, alter his form at will and therefore may appear slightly differently to different disciples. In Yogananda's descriptions he bears an uncanny resemblance to a young Lahiri Mahasaya. It is ultimately to Babaji that Yogananda attributes the revelation of "the possibility of bodily immortality."[55]

An account by Ram Gopal Muzumdar, as retold in the *Autobiography*, features not only Babaji but also his sister Mataji, who is alleged to be almost as spiritually advanced as her brother and remains in constant ecstasy in a secret underground cave near Dasaswamedh Ghat in Varanasi. Unlike his sister, Babaji is apparently more mobile and is thus purported to be ever wandering among the peaks of the Himalayas with a small band of disciples, which notably includes two very spiritually advanced Americans. In Muzumdar's account, Mataji uncharacteristically levitates out of her cave in a halo of light and is soon joined by her brother, who arrives in an airborne flaming whirlpool. Babaji, it turns out, has been thinking of shedding his form in order to return to the "Infinite Current." His sister seems unimpressed with this idea and inquires why he would leave his body. When Babaji asks what difference it makes if he "wear[s] a visible or an invisible wave on the ocean of [his] Spirit," Mataji points out that if it makes no difference, then he might as well keep his form.[56] To this Babaji replies by vowing that he will never henceforth leave his material body, always remaining visible to at least a small number of disciples on earth. Thus, the case of Babaji establishes fully divinized bodily immortality as a possibility alongside that of traditional notions of final liberation. It is important to note that Babaji's body, even though visibly resembling a physical human form, nevertheless exists entirely outside of the schema of conventional material embodiment as it is not held together by desire but by divine will.

We return thus to the dual model of yogic goals with which we began this study. This is Sarbacker's distinction of the numinous and the cessative all over again. However, in Yogananda's model, we see that the two are not only equally valued but interchangeable. Yogananda's own terminology somewhat belies this fact. After all, why would one choose to be anything other than supremely free? From one perspective, it appears that Babaji is making a bodhisattva-style sacrifice. He remains embodied for the sake of his disciples. However, Babaji himself maintains that it makes no difference—he is but a wave on the ocean of the absolute and whether that wave is visible or invisible (that is, with or without form) is largely beside the point. From a non-enlightened being's point of view, however, this distinction makes all the difference in the world. On the one hand, we have a walking, talking, fire-ball levitating Babaji and on the other we have . . . nothing. The impersonal universe.

The subtle undergirding of Yogananda's narrative, especially where it concerns his fascination with superpowers, is specifically a struggle with this distinction. When Sri Yukteswar bestows upon him a vision of the undifferentiated bliss of *samādhi*, he nevertheless persists in petulantly asking when he might acquire the miraculous powers that are, in his mind, equated with having found God. While there is an unmistakable tinge of monism throughout Yogananda's writings, it is at every turn balanced with the prospect of superhuman embodiment. One suspects that Yogananda's personal theology is very much based on the ultimate divinization of the human self. His reinterpretation of the nature of *avatāric* descent is testament to this. Although it appears nowhere in the *Autobiography*, he would frequently insist to his disciples that Babaji was in fact Krishna in a former incarnation.[57] This does not seem terribly earth-shattering until one combines it with the parallel proposition that Babaji started out human. In response to White's chicken-or-egg question[58] of whether Yogis are modeled on the gods, or the gods on Yogis, Yogananda would almost certainly have asserted the latter.

This prospect presents an interesting possibility. According to Yogananda, the science of Kriya Yoga is not so much a reagent as it is a catalyst or simply an accelerant. That is, the practice is not a necessary condition without which this process of spiritual evolution would be impossible. Rather, it serves to significantly accelerate an already ongoing natural process. From a narrative standpoint, Babaji's origins are never revealed (and the generic title Babaji is used as a familial honorific often ascribed to renunciants) precisely because Babaji's particular identity does not matter. He is the Everyman par excellence. In Yogananda's own words, Babaji is the proof of the possibility of human immortality and therefore of the final telos of the human as superhuman. Insomuch as we are all potential Yogis, we are also all Babaji.

Epilogue

I'm beyond Superman. . . . Because I have balls like atom
bombs, two of them, 100 megatons each. Nobody fucks
with me.

—BIKRAM CHOUDHURY

IT MIGHT BE said that Yogananda's death in 1952 marked the end of the first
wave of Indian-American Yogis. He arrived on Western shores in 1920 when
Americans were only beginning to recognize Yogis as anything more than cari-
catures in Oriental narratives. In some ways, the persona that Yogananda found
himself performing for his American audiences was profoundly consistent with
the persona of the Yogi as it had developed through millennia of Indian history.
The Yogi was still the man with superpowers. However, these superpowers were
increasingly articulated in ways that left behind ancient esoteric roots in favor of
a modern discourse of scientific rationalism. By the time that Yogananda took
up the title in America, the Theosophists and other Yogis like Vivekananda had
established a model of the Yogi as a universal ideal of superhumanity and the
exemplar of a natural process of human spiritual evolution.

Thus, not all Yogis of the time were Indian. However, Yogis who happened
to be Indian were far more vulnerable than their Western counterparts to the
negative racial stereotyping and exoticized expectations that the title evoked.
Yogananda, who had himself been fascinated since childhood by yogic superpowers, took to performing these superpowers in vaudeville productions that
must have at times felt only tangentially related to his loftier spiritual aspirations.
He was exoticized, feminized, villainized, and apotheosized by his audiences,
detractors, and devotees. In the meantime, he managed to create a system of
psycho-spiritual development that syncretized with impressive innovation traditional yogic and emerging Western metaphysical techniques and worldviews.

Ultimately, Yogananda's *Autobiography* is perhaps the best testament to the
deeply ambivalent nature of his identity and life's work. It conceals as much as it
reveals. And yet, in concealing, it reveals still more. Yogananda's conception of
the Yogi, problematized as it already was by traditional Indian folk conceptions

and colonial representations, could hardly have entirely prepared him for the role he would have to play as a South Asian immigrant-cum-exotic Oriental mystic as he navigated the political, social, and spiritual currents of the pre–World War II United States. Despite the many other reasons he might have had for largely glossing over his three decades in the West when he sat down to write the story of his life—from considerations of a popular audience thirsty for tales from the "Land of Miracles" to his personal investment in his identity as a Yogi and the concomitant relationship to his spiritual guru—one suspects that Yogananda may have chosen to omit these years because he did not quite know how to make sense of them.

There is something a bit sad about this aspect of the *Autobiography*. As dazzling as Yogananda's accounts of India continue to appear even upon his return, the all-too-brief homecoming leaves something unsaid. The death of his guru during this time, though historically accurate, is also metaphorically fitting. The American Yogi could not go home again. When Yogananda envisions the story of himself as a Yogi, that story resides in the myth of a spiritual India rather than in the considerable accomplishments of his work in the West.

All editions of the *Autobiography*, however, end with the same phrase: "Lord . . . Thou hast given this monk a large family!" At the end of his life, Yogananda envisioned himself as a "world citizen" just as the Yogi had become for him a universal ideal. Although yogic superpowers might have properly resided for him in mystic India, the science of yoga and the cosmic ideal of the superhuman Yogi knew no geographic bounds.

* * *

FAST FORWARD TWENTY-FIVE years. In a late-1970s American television segment,[1] a young Bikram Choudhury, clad in a black Speedo, white tube socks, and draped in a bright yellow polyester robe, drops an apple onto a bed of nails—the same bed of nails that only minutes later will support his body as another member of the "High Yogi Troupe of Calcutta" drives a motorcycle over a wooden ramp resting on his chest. The camera zooms in as an assistant guides Choudhury through a breathing exercise in preparation for what the voiceover commentary describes as "a very dangerous test of yoga philosophy." To the amazement of all, "Yogi Bikram" emerges unscathed, having demonstrated his perfect control over the "mental, physical, and spiritual forces" involved. Choudhury's senior students, who were either on the scene or witnesses to the aftermath, tell a slightly different story. The force of the motorcycle cracked Choudhury's head against the pavement, rendering him unconscious. He walked around with black holes dotting his back for weeks.[2] The television audience, of course, sees none of this. The footage cuts directly to Choudhury bounding up from his bed of nails like the superhuman Yogi he is touted to be.

The man driving the motorbike is Biswanath Ghosh, nephew of Paramahansa Yogananda and son of Bishnu Ghosh.

This young "sideshow" Bikram, with his tiny Speedo and his bed of nails, is the perfect contemporary incarnation of the Yogi ascetic. Four decades later, the picture is even more iconographically mind-boggling: Choudhury, the founder of Bikram Yoga, teaches his classes clad in his signature Speedo (now often leopard-print) and a diamond-encrusted Rolex, managing to evoke the ascetic-turned-capitalist Maharaja. In the figure of Bikram Choudhury, we encounter a sort of postmodern Yogi—a superman who eats a single meal a day (chicken or beef only), drinks nothing but water and Coke, and needs only two hours of sleep per night.[3] Indeed, through a complex set of calculations that account for the time an average human being spends sleeping, Choudhury has determined that he is approximately 220 years old.[4]

As it is commonly recounted, Choudhury's biography is really more of an auto-hagiography in its own right, except that his miracles usually involve curing celebrities and inventing the disco ball. When not in his teaching uniform, Choudhury adopts the style of Michael Jackson's glimmering gangster, codified somewhere between "Billie Jean" (1982) and "Smooth Criminal" (1987), which seems fair given that Choudhury claims to have launched Jackson's career. Benjamin Lorr, in his memoir-cum-ethnography of the competitive Bikram Yoga community, reports having stood behind Choudhury "when he thought he was off-mic and heard him muttering to himself over and over that he is 'Bikram, a gangster like Cagney, like De Niro, like James Caan, like my most favorite Mr. James Caan, Sonny Sonny Sonny Sonny Boy' while rubbing his hands and cackling to himself." This seems like an unethically personal detail to reveal, except that Lorr claims to have heard the same speech broadcast to an audience of hundreds on several other occasions.[5] Choudhury's behavior would seem insane if it were not so effective. His persona is a study in self-invention.

Here is yet another story. Bikram Choudhury was born in Calcutta in 1946.[6] We know little about his parents, except that they were the exacting type and threw their child into an intense yogic regimen at the tender age of three. He was handed over to Bishnu Ghosh, Yogananda's younger brother, soon thereafter—at the age of five or six, by most accounts. It was 1952, the same year that Yogananda took his final *samādhi*. Ghosh was by this time like a more finely muscled version of his older brother, performing superhuman feats that included stopping the heart, allowing an elephant to walk across his chest, and bending heavy iron bars. Under Ghosh, Choudhury's training intensified. He won the Indian National Yoga Competition at the age of thirteen and held the title, undefeated, for three years until he retired at the request of none other than the legendary B. K. S. Iyengar himself. After this he ran marathons, lifted weights, and reportedly engaged in all manner of superhuman exploits until, sometime between age seventeen and twenty, he dropped a 380-pound weight on his knee, shattering the patella. Doctors declared that he would never walk again, but Choudhury, refusing to go gentle into that good night, returned to his guru. Ghosh rebuilt him from the knees up with the miraculous yoga technology he had at his disposal. Through excruciating effort Choudhury emerged, a mere six months later, like the Six Million Dollar Man he was destined to become: better, stronger, faster.

After his rehabilitation, Choudhury left Calcutta to become the Yogiraj of Bombay, landing in Bollywood during the tail end of its "golden age." Today Bollywood films have become a staple of Choudhury's teacher training programs. He watches his stories into the early hours of the morning, fueling the legends of his sleeplessness. It was also during this period in Bombay that Choudhury first met the iconic American actress and New Age enthusiast Shirley MacLaine. MacLaine, like many spiritual seekers of her time, had come to live in India to find herself. Choudhury nevertheless told her, "You are in the wrong place. You won't find the truth in India. Go back to Hollywood, sing, dance and entertain the people; that's your duty, your Karma Yoga. When the time is right, India will come to you."[7]

Ghosh left his body in 1970 via what is reported to be a self-induced heart attack,[8] charging Choudhury to complete his brother Yogananda's mission of bringing yoga to the world. That same year, Choudhury left for Japan, where he introduced the use of a heated room to replicate the conditions of his native Calcutta, aided Japanese scientists studying tissue regeneration in publishing a series of papers, and healed a traveling Richard Nixon of chronic phlebitis using nothing but Epsom salts.[9] Some say that it was Nixon himself who invited Choudhury to America and met him on the runway, while others attribute the suggestion to MacLaine. Regardless, by 1973, Choudhury had made his way to California and opened a small school in Beverly Hills, where he quickly became yoga guru to the stars.

While Choudhury may have started out sleeping in the back room of his small Beverly Hills studio, four decades later he sleeps (or does not, as the case may be) in a sprawling mansion in the same locale. He has become famous for his diamond Rolexes and his fleet of Rolls-Royces. Gossip abounds regarding his harem of mistresses. In many ways, he is that mischaracterized Yogi described by the 1932 *Los Angeles Times* editorial with which we began this study—minus the turbans and snakes. His glitterati gangster persona calls up an interesting blend of old tropes: the fearsome *thuggee* (one of those marauding Yogi mercenaries), draped in Oriental luxe and updated to reflect the 1980s Hollywood that spawned Choudhury's yoga empire.

It is a well-known fact that in the twenty-first century, yoga has become big business.[10] While the previous chapters of this study have suggested that Yogis—and specifically American Yogis—have been deft entrepreneurs from the very start, it is Choudhury who was arguably among the first to instantiate yoga as a fully franchised, merchandized, and copyrightable product of consumer capitalism. He maintains that his efforts in this arena were prompted by MacLaine, who advised him that "in America, if you don't charge money . . . people won't respect you."[11] In 1994 Choudhury held his first open teacher training program at his Los Angeles location. At their peak in the early 2000s, his training programs would regularly boast upwards of 300 registrants.

Although his infamy had been steadily growing, Choudhury exploded into the mainstream media in 2002, when he filed a copyright infringement lawsuit against a group of yoga studios that were offering "Bikram Yoga" classes despite lacking formal certification from his organization. It was in part these efforts that prompted the Indian government to initiate the documentation of over 1,000 known yoga postures as part of the Traditional Knowledge Digital Library. Choudhury's lawsuit, which was challenged by a consortium of schools (several led by former senior teachers) under the title of Open Source Yoga Unity, was settled out of court under a non-disclosure agreement.[12] Choudhury's efforts have been marginally successful and the extent of his copyright continues to be contested. As Jordan Susman has observed at the culmination of a lengthy legal analysis of Choudhury's copyright claims:

> Had Bikram been more modest in his assertions and in his ambitions, he would have claimed that his sequence was an expressive dance and accentuated its aesthetic value. Although this might not have attracted huge throngs of followers, it would have afforded him maximum possible copyright protection. However, Bikram chose to be a savior—the man who developed the cure for all known illness.[13]

For Choudhury, it had to be both ways. He was both the owner of a commodity and the conduit of a universal system of salvific healing. Although it may be based on less than solid ground from a modern legal perspective, a closer examination of Choudhury's logic reveals something very interesting: his claim to ownership and the invocation of the copyright can easily be read as attempts to control a model of initiatory transmission through modern structures of economic and legal power.

In a 2014 press release responding to the continued phenomenon of studio owners offering something other than his authorized ninety-minute sequence, Choudhury proclaims:

Taking part in a pseudo-Bikram class is like having a nurse perform brain surgery. The only way to avoid unnecessary injuries is simple—stick to methods handed down by an original master. My system is endorsed by Bishnu Ghosh, my guru, who trained me in yoga's purest forms. He wanted to fulfill the mission of merging east and west begun last century by his brother, Paramahansa Yogananda, author of the classic *Autobiography of a Yogi*. While the message of Yogananda and others like him dwindles, my posture sequence has become part of the everyday lives of millions.[14]

This lineage is affirmed by the fact that the convocational meetings of Choudhury's teacher training programs take place in front of wreathed portraits of himself, Bishnu Ghosh, and Yogananda. The appeal to a lineage reveals a dimension of Choudhury's claims to power that transcends personal hubris. It also sheds new light on the logic behind his insistence that all of his teachers memorize a forty-five-page script (or "dialogue," as it is known in the community) that is meant to be recited verbatim. Every Bikram Yoga class must take place in a room designed according to a specific set of requirements, in a span of exactly ninety minutes, and contain a series of postures that is instructed in the same identical way every time. It is ritual action in its most basic form.

Moreover, it is my strong suspicion (though one that cannot be substantiated for obvious reasons) that Choudhury's twenty-six posture sequence may be the very sequence prescribed to him by Ghosh following his injury. My reasons for believing this are simple. First, the sequence is by no means holistic: it virtually ignores the upper body and the hips. Indeed, if one were to identify a primary focus—quickly corroborated by the effects on one's own body after a few months of regular practice—it is on the legs, and especially on the muscles surrounding the knees. Second, it is a sequence that can be performed by nearly anyone. That is its beauty. Even the weakest, the most unathletic, the most broken-down practitioner can perform these poses to some degree. Even someone who cannot stand. It would not be difficult to arrive at the conclusion that the reason Choudhury believes this practice is the only thing necessary to save a life is because it saved his. In this sense, every Bikram Yoga class becomes a reenactment of the sequence that saved, rebuilt, and transformed its founder. How's that for ritual?

The exact origins of the Bikram Yoga sequence aside, there is still something suggestive about the mechanics of its transmission. In Choudhury's own words, the purpose of the dialogue is to ensure that taking a class in any Bikram Yoga studio is in every way identical to taking a class from Choudhury himself. In other words, Choudhury is practicing, in a very real way, the ancient yogic superpower of tele-consciousness: through his dialogue, he very literally takes over the bodies and minds of others as conduits for his teaching. Just as the tantric guru ritually possesses the neophyte *sādhaka* as a mechanism of initiation, Choudhury infuses the minds of his teacher-trainees with his own transmission of clan knowledge.

If this seems farfetched, one need only spend a few months practicing Bikram Yoga. Choudhury's dialogue is recited by his teachers with remarkable consistency. After a while it creeps into your brain, unheeded, until you find yourself repeating it like yet another Bikram simulacrum, with its awkward grammar and its idiosyncratic phrasing— "Like a natural human traction . . . go back . . . way back . . . more back . . . fall back . . . change!" Seemingly opaque physical cues are internalized through embodied practice until they come to make perfect sense. Some reveal their foreign origins through references that the parroting teachers have no way of understanding as anything other than a turn of phrase. "L like Linda," Choudhury instructs his students, in a pose where they balance on one leg while forcefully kicking the other out in front of them. Linda was one of Choudhury's earliest students and one of his closest friends. They attended each other's weddings and raised their children together until things got "out of control" and she had to distance herself.[15] "L like Linda," say the teachers. To them Linda has become the right angle formed by the legs.

Through this practice, Choudhury has achieved as much immortality as may be possible without entering entirely into the realm of the superhuman. Every time a Bikram Yoga class is enacted, he is there. Of course, one wonders what will happen, as it does with many such communities, when his charismatic presence is no longer there to sustain the ritual. From a Weberian standpoint, the Yogi is the embodiment of charisma. Not the watered-down version used in daily conversation, but that electrifying preternatural kind. The kind that underlies conversion, or *śaktipat*, or makes people pass out in ecstatic sobs at music concerts.

Yet no matter how superhuman the Yogi becomes—or is believed by himself and by others to have become—the human encroaches. Great power brings great responsibility and the awesome can easily become the awful. We do not have access to premodern Indian *sādhakas*, or to Vivekananda, or to Yogananda, but we do have access to Bikram. The accusations that we saw played out in the trials of Pierre Bernard, both in the courtroom and the popular media, the allegations that dogged Yogananda's separations with two close friends and partners—these are now emerging in the enhanced access of the Internet age in the sexual assault charges leveled against Choudhury. To date several women have come forward alleging that Choudhury sexually assaulted them, often repeatedly, in the context of a power dynamic that can only be characterized as severely imbalanced. As I am putting the finishing touches on this manuscript, Choudhury has announced— mirroring Yogananda's post-Dhirananda-scandal move—that he will be returning to India.

And yet when we see Choudhury criticized for routinely comparing himself to Jesus Christ and the Buddha, we must remember that he is modeling himself on a legacy of earlier Yogis who were subjected to precisely such comparisons. The only difference is that these earlier Yogis generally did not apply such sobriquets to themselves—at least not in public—but allowed the media to act on their behalf. On the other hand, Yogananda was reportedly quite fond of claiming that he had been Arjuna and William the Conqueror in previous incarnations,[16] and disaffected disciples continue to claim that he impressed many a female student with tales of his valiant deeds.

Coda

Of course, most Bikram Yoga practitioners are not the least bit aware of their guru's implication in this lineage of the Yogi. Indeed, quite a few of them have no conception that "Bikram" is a real living person and not some foreign word that designates the style's ancient Indian origins. And yet, as Courtney Bender has argued, despite the general aversion to history shared by today's New Metaphysicals, practices do have memory.[17] Although, as Bender notes, "narrating spirituality in a way that gives it a past and affords it a tradition makes it unrecognizable to those who practice and produce it," a narrative of practice can help shed light on the ways in which spiritual identities are produced and reproduced. It is in this context that I will restate my original claim that what is key about the Yogi is not precisely who he is but what he does. In fact, it is what he does that makes him who he is. And what he does is embody, however tenuously, the possibility of the superhuman.

The performances of Yogananda, Ghosh, and Choudhury are in the final analysis not so different from the nineteenth-century strongmen and women who performed in vaudeville acts, bending iron bars and supporting seemingly impossible weights, or the contortionists who twisted themselves into equally impossible postures. Indeed, some of these performers were arguably more impressive than even the Yogi due to their theatrical inclinations. For instance, one Miss Darnett was famous for singing in a supine position as her chest and thighs supported a platform that held her musical accompaniment: a piano together with the pianist.[18] Decontextualized, such displays easily fall into the larger genre of freakery. The physically anomalous human body can inspire morbid fascination, as was the case with the early images of Yogi ascetics, but, framed correctly, it can also inspire wonder. There is a thin line within popular culture between the sideshow freak and the superhero.

The Yogi is significant insomuch as he provides a rich metaphysical precedent for the superhuman. With the introduction of the Theosophical Mahatmas and the subsequent rise of the Yogi mystic, the Yogi became an embodiment of universal human potential based on a complex metaphysical synthesis. From Nikola Tesla's short treatise on the implications of Vivekananda's metaphysics to Alan Moore's posthuman Doctor Manhattan with his suggestive blue hue and forehead markings, the twentieth century saw Indian referents consistently co-opted to construct Western models of the superhuman. The use of scientific language by pioneers of yoga in the West created an ideal context in which occult adepts could be made intelligible as scientifically perfected supermen.

In this context, the ostensibly magical powers of the Yogi transition from the realm of fantasy to something very much like science fiction. However, rather than rely on micro-elements of cognitive estrangement in the form of technologies or the new worlds they render accessible—though, as we saw, Yogananda's *Autobiography* offers something very much along these lines—the Yogi's metaphysics is a kind of macro "theory of everything" that expands the notion of the human individual into identity with the basic fabric of the universe.[19] Consequently, Joseph Alter has argued, "where the cyborg blurs natural boundaries and confuses categories, the yogi blurs the boundaries between biology, cosmology, and consciousness."[20]

In short, within the realm of twentieth-century American pop culture, the universalization (or de-Orientalization) and scientization of the Yogi figure create a space of slippage between the occult-spiritual (or fantastic) and the science fictional. Yogis give us a language to address the superhuman as a natural extension of scientific and evolutionary transhumanism. In this context, it seems like no coincidence that in the popular television serial *Heroes* (2006–1010), wherein a group of ordinary individuals suddenly discover that a genetic mutation has endowed them with a variety of superpowers, the doctor who originally posits the possibility of such an evolutionary outcome is Indian.[21]

The plot point seems random until one examines the pattern of such origin stories. Take, for instance, the central figure of the "Chandu the Magician" franchise, which ran as a popular radio show between 1931 and 1935, before being revived in 1948–50. The character was also featured in a motion-picture film and subsequent serial, *Chandu the Magician* (1932) and *The Return of Chandu* (1934), both starring the legendary Bela Lugosi, first as Chandu's arch nemesis Roxor and returning as Chandu himself. Unlike most early depictions of the Yogi, however, Chandu is distinguished by being a Westerner. Chandu, whose original name is Frank Chandler, is an American who travels to Tibet to learn Eastern magics from a Yogi master and returns endowed with superpowers that aid him through a myriad of mysteries and adventures.

Despite being an American, Chandu is depicted as the typical turbaned Yogi gazing into his crystal ball. The chief action of the first film notably revolves around his attempts to thwart the attempts of Roxor (who is himself an Egyptian mystic) to destroy the earth with a death-ray machine (fig. E.1). It is worth noting that the death-ray is a decidedly scientific apparatus, despite the fact that Roxor presumably has much more "mystical" means of destruction at his disposal. Indeed, the death-ray, which was actually first envisioned by Tesla as a technology of world peace,[22] would, along with the futurist engineer's other popular invention—the eponymous Tesla coil—would become a favorite staple of pop culture supervillains and mad scientists for decades to come. The story arch of a turbaned American Yogi poised against an Oriental mystic using Western technology is itself a testament to the increasingly blurry lines between not only the mystical and the scientific but the racialized Yogi and the "universalized" superman.

Then there is Chondu the Mystic, a Marvel comic book character who first appears in 1960 in the *Tales of Suspense* series as a sideshow magician at a carnival who lectures on yoga and the potential of the human mind and subsequently exhibits some superhuman abilities of his own. Chondu has no formal links to the earlier Chandu, aside from the fact that both appear as turbaned Westerners who share remarkably similar names. Chondu returns for a longer stint as a

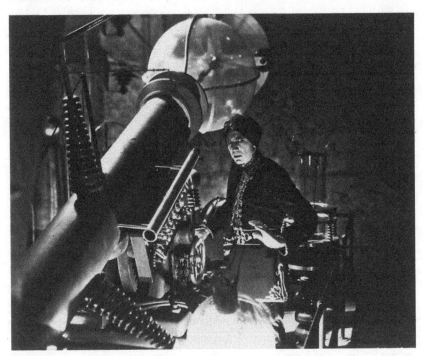

FIGURE E.1 Bela Lugosi as Roxor, the Egyptian mystic turned supervillain, with his death-ray machine in *Chandu the Magician* (1932)

supervillain and member of the Headmen in Marvel's *Defenders* series in 1975 and subsequently reprises this role in several more volumes. However, he quickly ceases to resemble any form that would identify him as a Yogi (in the traditional Orientalist sense) or even human—although the fact that his main narrative arc involves the transplantation of his head and/or consciousness on/into a variety of different bodies may well point to the traditional yogic ability to possess the bodies of others. If nothing else, the former Yogi is definitively no longer quite human. The original Chandu also ultimately served as inspiration for Marvel's Doctor Strange, who first appeared in *Strange Tales* #110 (1963) billed as the "Master of Black Magic." The character of Doctor Stephen Strange was subsequently developed as a brilliant neurosurgeon who, after a tragic car accident shatters his hands, journeys to the Himalayas to acquire superhuman abilities from a hermit known only as the Ancient One.

Finally, there is the aforementioned example of the blue-hued Doctor Manhattan, arguably the most "super" of the superheroes in Alan Moore's *Watchmen* (1986). As before, the genealogy misses a few links here, unless one considers the fact that in the late 1960s Doctor Strange received a short-lived makeover that turned him into a well-built blue humanoid.[23] While the Doctor Manhattan character is never formally linked to anything other than science (especially in his human form as Jon Osterman, the nuclear physicist), his blue superhuman form draws on a variety of occult and Indian religious elements. While not an explicit Yogi-figure, Doctor Manhattan illustrates the many levels of cultural imbrication between the occult and the scientific. He is, of course, named after the Manhattan Project, the ultimate product of which prompted another nuclear physicist named J. Robert Oppenheimer to quote one of the most famous Yogis of all when he said, "Now I am become Death, the destroyer of worlds."

Returning to Choudhury, if the rationale behind his sometimes outlandish claims is opaque to most practitioners of modern postural yoga, the narratives just described are even further removed from anything they would identify with their practice. Yet the historical connections are undeniable, and if one ever begins to wonder why Bikram Choudhury often resembles a manic comic book villain, the answers may lie precisely within this history.

By the time that World War II drew to a close, the Yogi had already begun to morph. The lecture circuit that had once been littered with Indian expatriate Yogis dried up as these individuals drew their careers to a natural close and no new ones came to take their place. The immigration regulations imposed in the 1920s yielded their intended outcome. As a result, yoga slowly began to fade into the generic landscape of New Thought, and the Yogi gradually became a Westerner who had traveled to India to acquire powers rather than the Indian himself.

The Yogi mystic of the prewar era became increasingly abstracted in his popular instantiations. Universalization is a powerful tool of propagation, but it also dilutes and erases.[24] In this case, the universalizing impulse had succeeded: the Yogi had become the superhuman Everyman, but in doing so he was recognizable as a Yogi only to those who knew to look for his mark in iconographic hints and origin stories.

The Immigration and Naturalization Act of 1965 changed all that. With the lifting of immigration quotas, a new wave of teachers was able to enter the United States, and American interest in yoga slowly began to reawaken. According to Bender:

> Yoga students and teachers alike heralded the arrival of Asian religious teachers as authentic and knowledgeable practitioners from the 1970's on as avatars of true yoga, thus displacing earlier forms and expressions as less than authentic and glossing over the longer histories of exchange that shape yoga in both India and the United States.[25]

This assertion is insightful, if a little overstated. As Bender herself notes, modern yoga practitioners, like most metaphysically inclined seekers, generally express no significant inclination toward historical inquiry. Even the more committed view their practice as the instantiation of a perennial wisdom, and thus questions of its synthesis during the early twentieth century hardly ignite the imagination. And yet the linkages are there, and today's communities of spandex-clad Yogis would hardly exist without the historical scaffolding that secured the yoga's place on the American landscape of therapeutic spirituality.

As Yogananda was propagating his updated form of *haṭha* yogic practice geared at a metaphysical body beautiful, a parallel synthesis was likewise well under way on the other side of the globe. Yogananda encountered one of the chief denizens of the Second Wave Yogis during his single return to India in 1936. There, while touring the south of the Indian subcontinent, he visited Krishnamacarya's Mysore Palace school and witnessed the postural acrobatics of one very young B. K. S. Iyengar, whom he promptly invited back to the United States.[26] One wonders what would have happened if Iyengar had agreed. What if Iyengar had been trained in Yogananda's lineage of *haṭha* yoga rather than Krishnamacarya's? What if he had come to the West a full quarter of a century earlier? Would Bikram Choudhury exist? Would his glimmering gangster suits, tiny Speedos, and novel form of postural practice still have captivated America? One suspects so. After all, as I have sought to demonstrate with respect to both Choudhury and Yogananda, a man who has determined himself to be a Yogi will seek to prevail despite all obstacles.

It is not common to hear modern Yogis promise their followers superpowers, as Yogananda had once done. Bikram Choudhury too is likely a dying breed. Today's Yogi icons, who are increasingly blonde and female, generally stop at promising toned bodies and the kind of spiritual fulfillment that feels like watching a sunset placidly melt into the California ocean. The Yogi's superpowers, in the meantime, have migrated into the superhero lore that serves as our modern-day mythology. From that perspective, it is not surprising that Ashok Kumar Malhotra's contribution to the Ashgate World Philosophies Series—entitled *An Annotated Introduction to Yoga Philosophy* (2001) but essentially comprising an annotated translation of the *Yoga Sūtras*—features an entire section on "Yoga and Yoda." The Jedi (*Jogi*. Yogi?) is the adept struggling with the lure of superpower, Darth Vader is the fallen master bound to his mortal body by his mechanized breathing, and Yoda is the wizened mystic who has become a wave on the ocean of the Force.[27]

If Yogananda's legacy teaches us only one thing, it is perhaps that the Yogiman is perpetually somewhere between the Bogeyman and Superman.

Notes

PREFACE

1. De Michelis 2004: 2.

INTRODUCTION

1. Yogananda 1926c: 15.
2. I use the currently accepted form of Yogananda's name and title. Until 1935, when he was awarded the title of Paramahansa (literally, "Supreme Swan," after the bird's legendary powers of discernment), he went by Swami Yogananda. After 1935, he billed himself as Paramhansa Yogananda, utilizing the phonetic spelling of the title. The Self-Realization Fellowship corrected the spelling to the proper Sanskrit "Paramahansa" after Yogananda's death, going so far as to insert the extra "a" into his signature as it adorns the covers of his books. I have preserved the original spelling in all relevant quotes and citations.
3. This statement does not include the several collected volumes that have appeared over the years addressing individual gurus who have visited or lived in the United States over the course of the previous century and their organizations. Although such texts offer useful case studies, they are generally limited in their scope and do not offer a sustained analysis beyond the biography of the specific individual in question. Such studies include Harper 1972; Copley 2000; Forsthoefel and Humes 2005; Singleton and Goldberg 2014; Gleig and Williamson 2014. Gleig and Williamson's volume focuses specifically on "homegrown" or European-American gurus.
4. See Jain 2014b.
5. White 2009: 45.
6. White 2009: 44–45.
7. White 2009: 175.

8. Siegel 2014: 28–35. Siegel particularly distinguishes between the powers of *vaśitva*, or mastery over one's own mind and being (one of the classic eight *siddhis*), and *vaśīkaraṇa*, or power over the minds of others. The latter particularly can be related to the traditional yogic talents of illusions, such as *yogamāyā* or *indrajāla*, and the more modern usage of *sammohan*, which more directly translates as hypnotism.

9. Pinch 2006: 16.

10. See Jain 2014b.

11. Sarbacker 2011: 198.

12. Pinch 2006: 66.

13. See especially DeMichelis 2004; Strauss 2005; Jain 2014a.

14. See, for instance, Hanegraaff 1996.

15. Albanese 2007: 13–15.

16. See Jacobsen 2011: 2. Jacobsen's volume as a whole offers a complex overview of the roles of supernatural powers in a variety of yogic traditions.

17. This usage is briefly adopted in Kripal 2011: 172.

18. Although the first explosion of American superhero narratives does not properly come until the 1930s, these characters thereafter absorb and appropriate much from the mystic powers associated with the Yogi. See, for instance, Kripal 2011: 171–72; 211–16.

19. Vivekananda 1915: 142.

20. "Fakir" tends to appear more frequently when the tone is derogatory and was indeed fairly common in contemporaneous parlance and often suggestively pronounced as "faker." For a more complex analysis and the more positive valences held by the term, see Dobe 2015.

21. Iwamura 2011: 6.

22. Said 1978: 3.

23. Iwamura 2011: 9.

24. Isaacs 1958: 29.

25. Isaacs 1958: 45.

26. Singer 1972: 21.

27. Pollock 1993.

28. King 1999: 93.

29. King 1999: 97.

30. See Dehejia 1986 and White 2002.

31. Although female practitioners are instrumental to key tantric ritual practices, the scholarship on such traditions has viewed these women as just that—instruments or assistants present to complement male practice but rarely having much agency of their own. There are some notable exceptions to this within the scholarship of Miranda Shaw (1995) and Loriliai Biernacki (2007), but the overwhelming trend is clear.

32. See White 1996 and 2002.

33. Alter 2011a: 127
34. See O'Flaherty 1981.
35. Lee 1999: 85.
36. See De Michelis 2004.
37. See Love 2010; Laycock 2013; Jain 2014b.
38. Stephens 2010: 24. I take Stephens's use of "bhakti," "raja," and "Hatha" to correspond to devotional, meditative, and postural practice, respectively.
39. Gandhi 2009: 38.
40. See especially Singleton 2005, 2007, 2010.
41. See Nance 2009.
42. See Williamson 2010.
43. Vivekananda arrived in the United States in 1893 and delivered public and private lectures around the country, returning to India in early 1897. During this time, he made two brief visits to the United Kingdom in 1895 and 1896.
44. Kriyananda was born James Donald Walters in 1926. He became Yogananda's disciple in 1948 after reading the *Autobiography* and remained with the SRF until 1962 when the board of directors voted unanimously in favor of his resignation for reasons that are still contested.
45. See Goldberg 2010: 109.
46. Rinehart 1999.
47. Leeman and di Florio 2014.
48. Shontell 2013.

CHAPTER 1

1. Oman 1903: 173.
2. On this point, see especially White 2014. In the context of modern postural yoga, the *Yoga Sūtras* are still idealized as the canon of "true" classical practice. However, the disjunction with practical reality remains: the meditative methodology of the text is just as at odds with today's athletic practice as it is with early modern conceptions of the habits of Yogis.
3. Pinch 2006: 6.
4. Isaacs 1958: 259.
5. Holdrege 1996: 230.
6. White 2009: 100.
7. White 2009: 96.
8. See Sarbacker 2005.
9. As evidenced by the breadth of essays in Jacobsen 2011.
10. Hatley 2007: 363–64.
11. See Ernst 2003 and 2005.
12. See Torzsok 1999 and Brunner 1975.

13. It is worth pointing out that Yogananda refers to just such a Yogi in his *Autobiography* when he recounts the story of "A Mohammedan Wonder-Worker" (chapter 18), a fakir who gained control over a "disembodied spirit" called Hazrat.

14. Rastelli 2000: 358–59.

15. Brunner 1975: 434–35.

16. White 2009: 168.

17. Lamont 2004: 3–4. See also White 2009: 207–8.

18. See White 2009 and Pinch 2006.

19. Bernier 1976: 316–21.

20. For an account of such performances in the context of Indian street magic, see Siegel 1991.

21. White 2009: 200–201.

22. See Diamond 2013: 236–57.

23. See Narayan 1993.

24. Oman 1903: 26–27.

25. Rose 1916: 289.

26. Lamont 2004: 20.

27. See Lamont 2004 and Siegel 1991.

28. Lamont 2004: 30.

29. Lamont 2004: 30–31.

30. See Lamont 2004 for an extensive history of the Indian rope trick. The majority of the subsequent account draws on his work.

31. See Lamont 2004: 159.

32. Lamont 2004: 80–81.

33. Lamont 2004: 82.

34. See Altman 2013 for a more complex account of the construction and representation of Hinduism prior to this period.

35. Quoted in Syman 2010: 16.

36. Thoreau 2004: 48–51.

37. Syman 2010: 33.

38. Syman 2010: 29.

39. "Thoreau" in *Fraser Magazine*, reprinted in *Eclectic Magazine* on August 1866, p. 180. Quoted in Syman 2010: 26.

40. See King 1999: 7–35, 118–43.

41. The publication on Arnold's work in England also coincided with the founding on the Pali Text Society in 1881 by Thomas William Rhys Davids. Rhys Davids, who first became familiar with Buddhist literature as a civil servant in colonial British India, went on to serve as Professor of Pali at the University of London from 1882 to 1904. He advocated for the nobility and pristine origins of Buddhism based partially on a racialized Aryan identity that formed a common bond between Britain and the Buddha's own kingdom. Many of these points were published in his

Lectures on the Origin and Growth of Religion as Illustrated by Some Points in the History of Indian Buddhism (1881).

42. Arnold 1879: 84–85.
43. Arnold 1879: 119.
44. Oman 1889: 47.
45. Ramacharaka 1903: 4.
46. Burke 1958: 10.
47. De Michelis 2004: 97.
48. Sil 1997: 27
49. See Sil 1997: 41–49 and De Michelis 2004: 100–108.
50. Sil 1997: 41–49.
51. De Michelis 2004: 105.
52. Sil 1997: 121.
53. Syman 2010: 38.
54. Atulananda 1938: 60.
55. Quoted in Sil 1997: 129.
56. Josephine MacLeod in 1895, quoted in Sil 1997: 93.
57. Quoted in Burke 1958: 28.
58. Burke 1958: 29.
59. Quoted in Sil 1997: 93.
60. Sil 1997: 21.
61. 1894 letter, quoted in Sil 1997: 116.
62. Sil 1997: 117.
63. Burke 1958: 211.
64. Vivekananda 1989b: 326.
65. Sil 1997: 169.
66. Sil 1997: 142.
67. Sil 1997: 87.
68. Syman 2010: 69–70.
69. Abhedananda 1902: 50.
70. Abhedananda 1902: 49.
71. Abhedananda 1902: 49.
72. See Alter 2014.
73. See Lal and Prasad 1999: 42–48.
74. Sohi 2014: 14–15.
75. Bald 2013: 7–9, 11–48.
76. Howard 1974.
77. Deslippe 2015 establishes that a transnational lecture circuit created a strong network not only along the coastal United States but also throughout the Midwest.
78. Wassan 1939: 359–79.

79. For an analysis of the intersection of tantra and Western Esotericism, see Urban 2003.
80. Quoted in Syman 2010: 97.
81. *Los Angeles Times* 1919. Also quoted in Syman 2010: 82.
82. For a more elaborate account of Westerners "playing Oriental," see Nance 2009.
83. See Kramer 2011.
84. Cullen et al. 2007: 580. See also Deslippe 2014. For an analysis of Yogis, "Hindoos," and racial passing, see Rocklin 2016 and Bald 2013: 49–93.
85. See Prothero 2004: 13–14.
86. *Chicago Daily Tribune* 1911.
87. Prothero 2004: 17.
88. *New York Times* 1909.
89. *Los Angeles Times* 1910.
90. *Los Angeles Times* 1926.
91. Adams 1935: 1.
92. *Washington Post* 1910.
93. See, for instance, Bednarowski 1980; Wessinger 1993; and Braude 2001.
94. See Love 2010: 76–77.
95. Reed 1914: 117.
96. Reed 1914: 131.
97. Reed 1914: 129.
98. Reed 1914: 131.
99. Gross Alexander is the author's husband. Her proper first name is not available, which is perhaps telling in itself.
100. See Jain 2014a: 23–24 and Schmidt 2010.

CHAPTER 2

1. See, for instance, Moore 1977 and Carroll 1997 for a treatment of the features, widespread popularity, and ideological implications of American Spiritualism.
2. On the subject of the diffuse nature of mind cure ideology as concerning the harmonial religious but also secular psychological spheres, see Meyer 1965.
3. Burke 1958: 211.
4. See Singleton 2007b: 125–46. Of course, Indian religious history is itself replete with traditions centered on the ritual perfection of the human body and the broader ideologies behind these are surely not to be discounted when examining the Indian origins of modern yoga or the figure of the Yogi.
5. Heelas 1996.
6. Trine 1897: 18.
7. See Albanese 2007.
8. Albanese 1999: 307–8.

9. This might seem like a tempting premise for the models of *ākāśa* as the all-pervading and eternal ground of materiality developed by the Theosophists and Vivekananda, except that in Nyāya-Vaiśeṣika *ākāśa* possesses no creative faculty. Indeed, unlike the other *mahābhūta*s, it can be considered eternal specifically because it does not consist of parts and cannot form aggregates. The eternality of *ākāśa* in Nyāya-Vaiśeṣika is specifically owed to its status as the substratum of sound (*śabda*), the corresponding eternality of which holds theological significance due to the significance attributed by these schools to the language of the Vedas.

10. Later commentators wrestle with these particularities. For instance, in the eighth century, the monistically inclined philosopher Śaṃkara catalogues several different philosophical arguments concerning the cosmic nature and all-pervasiveness of *ākāśa* before asserting that it must nevertheless be created and fundamentally different from the ultimate monistic reality of Brahman, constituting instead the first material evolute (Duquette and Ramasubramanian 2010: 521–24). Alternatively, in a sixteenth-century commentary on Sāṃkhya (*Sāṃkhyapravacanabhāṣya*), Vijñānabhikṣu asserts that there exist two kinds of *ākāśa*: the elemental *kāryākāśa*, which is atomic and non-eternal, and the causal *kāraṇākāśa*, which is non-atomic and gives rise to the all-pervasive categories of space (*diś*) and time (*kāla*) that characterize *prakṛti*'s potential changeability. However, this distinction does not appear in classical Sāṃkhya, nor is it particularly representative of the commentarial tradition at large.

11. White 1996: 210–12 and 241–43. Here, the chief significance of ether (whatever the Sanskrit term used) is that it is associated with the qualities of a void and therefore literally provides space for the tantric practitioner to concentrate his meditative practice.

12. Cantor and Hodge 1981: 4.

13. Cantor and Hodge 1981: 6. Interestingly, ether plays no major role in the Hermetic textual corpus—a synthesis of Stoic, Platonic, Judaic, and Christian strains of thought most likely arising in Alexandria during the first three centuries of the Common Era—which is universally acknowledged as a major originating current of modern metaphysical traditions. An honorable mention goes to the Latin *Asclepius* text (not generally dated and thought to be the remnant of an earlier Greek version), where *aether* is cited as generating the form of intellect unique to man (Cantor and Hodge 1981: 9). Otherwise, the semi-material substance, often referred to as the "quint-essence," would continue to appear in Christian theological writings whenever an ideological bridge between the realms of matter and spirit was deemed necessary, but its nature generally remained unelaborated.

14. Cantor and Hodge 1981: 12.

15. Cantor and Hodge 1981: 14.

16. Cantor and Hodge 1981: 22.

17. Cantor and Hodge 1981: 22–23.

18. James Clerk Maxwell's famous set of equations, which form the basis of modern electrodynamics, demonstrated in 1862 that light was an electromagnetic wave identical to heat. An ethereal fluid thus became even further entrenched as the unique form of matter required for the propagation of these waves. Because light is capable of traveling even through a vacuum, it was hypothesized that even such spaces must be filled with a non-moving ethereal substance. The first moment of crisis came in 1887 when the now famous Michelson-Morley experiment, conducted by Albert Michelson and Edward Morley, which attempted to measure the relative motion of matter through the stationary luminiferous ether, returned a null result. More specifically, the experiment was designed to measure the "ethereal wind" that would result from the earth and ether being in relative motion. However, it failed to detect any significant change in the relative speed of light that would have indicated a change in the motion of the earth in relation to the ether. Several subsequent experiments attempted to measure the effects of the ether's presence but returned no valid results, suggesting that a new theory was needed to account for the propagation of electromagnetic waves without the presence of a material medium.

19. These should be understood in addition to and, to a certain extent, in the context of the many other nearly identical theorized forms of a subtle universal substance, both scientific and occult. Notable mentions include Baron Karl Ludwig von Reichenbach's (1788–1869) "Odic Force" and Edward Bulwer-Lytton's (1803–1873) "Vril."

20. The second major point in Mesmer's theory, as explained in *Reflections on the Discovery of Animal Magnetism* (1779), quoted in Fuller 1982: 5.

21. Fuller 1982: 7.

22. See Crabtree 1993.

23. Blavatsky 1980: 220.

24. Kriyananda 2011: 267–68.

25. The phrase actually originates from *Thought Vibration or the Law of Attraction in the Thought World* (1906), penned by William Walter Atkinson who also wrote under the famous pseudonym of Yogi Ramacharaka.

26. Albanese 2007: 195.

27. Albanese 2007: 198. See also Jung-Stilling and Jackson 1844.

28. Albanese 2007: 199–204.

29. Kate and Margaret Fox, respectively, twelve and fifteen years old at the time, first heard mysterious rappings at their parents' home in Hydesville, New York, in 1848. They attributed the rappings to a spirit, to whom they referred as Mr. Splitfoot. The two girls would go on to become popular Spiritualist mediums and this incident is generally identified by historians as the start of the nineteenth-century Spiritualist movement at large.

30. Raia 2007: 38; Brain 2013: 120.

31. Brain 2013: 116.

32. Noakes 2007.

33. Most studies of Spiritualism make at least brief mention of ways in which medium-
    ship was instrumental in creating a space for women in the public sphere generally
    and as spiritually authoritative agents more particularly. See especially Braude 2001.

34. See Horowitz 2009: 69–74.

35. Olcott 1875: x.

36. Olcott 1875: 453.

37. Blavatsky 1969: 543.

38. Campbell 1980: 29.

39. Blavatsky 1966: 244.

40. Blavatsky 1954: 239.

41. Report of the committee of the Society of Psychical Research, quoted in Campbell
    1980: 93.

42. Ellwood 1979: 56.

43. There is no official membership data available prior to 1907, though the number of
    charters issued to lodges steadily increases during the years following the Society's
    inception to 913 in 1906, though it should be noted that this figure does not reflect
    the number of actually operational lodges at that time. As of 1907, the Society
    boasted an international membership of 14,863 persons with the highest minority
    of that number (4,548) being concentrated in India.

44. De Michelis 2004: 69–71. See also Van der Veer 2001: 55–82.

45. De Michelis 2004: 69–71.

46. Vivekananda 1915: 154.

47. Vivekananda 1966: 318–19.

48. Vivekananda 1915: 167.

49. See De Michelis 2004: 150.

50. Blavatsky 1877: 134.

51. Ultimately he is forced to admit that "both Akasha and Prana again are produced
    from the cosmic Mahat, the Universal Mind, the Brahmâ or Ishvara." See Swami
    Vivekananda, *The Complete Works*, 5:lvii. Of course, this is hardly any less prob-
    lematic, since it essentially takes *mahat* (or *buddhi*) out of its proper place in the
    schema of subtle materiality while simultaneously misidentifying it with the uni-
    versal Brahman.

52. De Michelis 2004: 157.

53. Jackson 1994: 75.

54. Vivekananda 1989b: 172.

55. Vivekananda 1989a: 78.

56. Raia 2007; Noakes 2008.

57. See Asprem 2014: 208–25.

58. Stewart and Tait 1875: 147.

59. Stewart and Tait 1875: 145.

60. Stewart and Tait 1875: 148.

61. Tesla 2011: xvi.
62. Tesla 2011: 80.
63. Tesla 1930.
64. Tesla 1930.
65. Vivekananda 1915: 167.
66. Vivekananda 1915: 182.
67. Vivekananda 1915: 264–65.
68. Einstein 1920.
69. See Albanese 1999.
70. Albanese 1999: 311.
71. Sinclair 1962: 133. Interestingly, later editions of Sinclair's work feature a short—
    and admittedly lukewarm—preface by Einstein. The physicist was a family friend
    of the Sinclairs, and even once attended a demonstration by the stage magician
    cum mystic Roman Ostoja at their home, so one might choose to read an amount
    of familiar indulgence into his testimony. Nevertheless, he concludes that though
    Sinclair's experiments "stand surely far beyond those which a nature investiga-
    tor holds to be thinkable," Sinclair's character demands that "in no case should
    the psychologically interested circles pass over this book heedlessly" (Sinclair
    1962: ix).
72. Yogananda 1951: 134.
73. Yogananda 1986: 132–33.
74. Yogananda 1951: 264.
75. Yogananda 1951: 235.
76. Yogananda 1999: 921. Yogananda is quoted as describing *akāśa* as "the subtle back-
    ground against which everything in the universe becomes perceptible. . . . space
    gives dimension to objects; ether separates the images" (Yogananda 1999: 867n).
77. Yogananda 1951: 42.
78. Yogananda 1951: 42.
79. Yogananda 1951: 242.
80. Yogananda 1951: 237.
81. Yogananda 1951: 237–38.
82. For a traditional reading of the physics of yogic power, see White 1984: 55–56.
83. Yogananda 1951: 238.
84. Yogananda 1951: 279.
85. Such an advertisement appeared in *The Los Angeles Times* on January 6, 1925.

CHAPTER 3

1. Davis 2006: 28–29.
2. Warnack 1932: 19.
3. For instance, Satyeswarananda quotes on multiple occasions and otherwise references Yogananda's work, most notably when he criticizes the multiple organizations

that Yogananda founded as well as Yogananda's subsequent mismanagement of them.

4. See Satyananda 2004. Yogananda cites much of his account as being translated from the Bengali edition of Satyananda's biography.

5. Satyeswarananda 1983: 217.

6. See Mallinson 2006. A more complete account of Kriya Yoga practice is offered in chapter 4.

7. Sri Yukteswar's full monastic name is Swami Sriyukteswar Giri, the "Sri" actually comprising a portion of his name rather than an honorific, as might be assumed. He was given the name upon taking his vows due to his habit of addressing attendants at his ashram with the traditional honorifics Sriyukta and Srimati rather than their anglicized equivalents (see Satyananda 2004: 53). Consequently, abbreviating the Swami's name to simply "Yukteswar," as is sometimes done, is technically incorrect. However, for the sake of recognizability, I have chosen to render his name as two separate units—Sri Yukteswar—as Yogananda does.

8. Satyeswarananda 1985: 44.

9. Satyeswarananda 1985: 45.

10. A circular group dance based in the mythology of Kṛṣṇa-Gopāla, or the god Krishna in his cowherd form.

11. Satyeswarananda 1985: 46; Satyananda 2004: 62.

12. These events are described in detail in chapter 2 of the *Autobiography*.

13. This presumably refers to the "hardcore" variety of tantra involving sexual rituals and impure substances. Kriya Yoga is itself a decidedly tantric practice, albeit of the internalized "softcore" variety.

14. Satyananda 2004: 169.

15. Satyananda 2004: 172.

16. See Esdaile 1846. For an exploration of the relationship between Indian and Western notions of hypnotism, including Esdaile's own role, see Siegel 2014.

17. "*Sammohan*," when it appears in Hindi or Bengali, tends usually to be translated as "hypnotism" and associated with *vaśya* or *vaśitva siddhi* (the power to subjugate others to one's will) among the classical list of the eight primary *siddhis*.

18. Ghosh 1980: 122–23.

19. Ghosh 1980: 125–26.

20. Mediumistic possession is not as common in the Indian context as other types, but does occasionally appear under the name of *svasthāveśa*, where voluntary or invited possession by deities and/or mid-level spirits is effected for the purposes of divination, especially upon a child (see Smith 2006: 416ff).

21. Yogananda 1946: 50.

22. Satyananda 2004: 159.

23. Not to be confused with Dayananda Saraswati, founder of the Ārya Samāj.

24. Ghosh 1980: 156.

25. Satyeswarananda 1985: 109.
26. Satyeswarananda 1991: 150.
27. Satyeswarananda 1994: 99.
28. Satyeswarananda 1994: 101.
29. Satyeswarananda 1994: 92.
30. Thomas 1930: 140–41.
31. Dhirananda's *Philosophic Insight* (1926) is advertised as available for purchase in a bundle along with four of Yogananda's books. Presumably this would not have been the case after 1929, when Dhirananda broke with Yogananda.
32. See Rosser 1991.
33. Satyananda 2004: 264.
34. Walters 2004: 77.
35. Satyeswarananda 1994: 108.
36. Choudhury 2007: 32.
37. Walters 2004: 91.
38. *New York Times* 1928.
39. *Miami Daily News* 1928b.
40. *Miami Daily News* 1928a.
41. *Miami Daily News* 1928b.
42. *Los Angeles Times* 1928.
43. *Los Angeles Times* 1935a.
44. *Los Angeles Times* 1935b.
45. Swami Giri-Dhirananda, also known as Basu Kumar Bagchi v. Swami Yogananda, also known as Mukunda Lal Ghosh, No. 387391 (Cal. Super. Ct. 1935).
46. *Los Angeles Times* 1939.
47. *Los Angeles Times* 1940b.
48. *Los Angeles Times* 1940a.
49. Walters 2004: 197.
50. Charlton 1990: 78. Hilda Charlton met Yogananda at a small lecture in Santa Barbara and briefly stayed with him in Encinitas and then at Mt. Washington. She ultimately left without becoming disciple, though later received Yogananda's mail-order lessons.
51. Kriyananda 2011: 266.
52. Rosser 1991: 48.
53. Charlton 1990: 96.
54. Charlton 1990: 97. Yogananda also performed the "six men" demonstration in Boston (see Kriyananda 2011: 35).
55. *Los Angeles Times* 1923.
56. *New York Times* 1927.
57. Yogananda 1927: 23–24.
58. Sinclair's *Mental Radio* (1931) does allude to the fact that Ostoja had had to travel all the way to India to acquire his skills, but this appears only as an incidental aside.

59. Satyeswarananda 1991: 150.
60. Satyananda 2004: 268.
61. Trout 2000: 120.
62. Satyeswarananda 1994: 115.
63. Satyeswarananda 1991: 149.
64. Dasgupta 2006: 121.
65. Dasgupta 2006: 132.
66. See Angel 1994: 293–96.
67. Yogananda 1958: 124.

CHAPTER 4

1. Warnack 1932: 19.
2. The most notable point of divergence, aside from the eschewing of Sanskrit terminology and exclusion of karma yoga, is Yogananda's subdivision of Vivekananda's
   rāja yoga into what he calls the "meditation method" and the "organic scientific
   method." The two new methods differ in that the "meditation method" is described
   as referring simply to the control of the external organs and is therefore judged to be
   hardly superior to the state of deep sleep. On the other hand, the "organic, scientific
   method," which receives a much lengthier exposition, deals with the control of the
   internal organs and life energies. This latter approach largely mirrors Vivekananda's
   description of *rāja yoga*, as well as the principles that would later guide Yogoda
   methodology as expounded by Yogananda, in combining a *haṭha* yogic physiology
   with scientific language of electromagnetism. The book is also composed in a lofty
   philosophical style that is highly uncharacteristic of Yogananda's later publications,
   one possible explanation for which is that Yogananda was not in fact the "instrumental cause" of the publication. In the preface to his "rewriting" of the work, *God
   Is for Everyone* (2003), Kriyananda claims that Yogananda never really wrote *The
   Science of Religion* at all. According to Laurie Pratt (Tara Mata), Yogananda drew
   up the outline for the book after his return from Japan in 1916 but Dhirananda,
   whose command of English was then far superior, served as a ghostwriter for the
   actual text. Dhirananda is listed as a secondary author on every edition of the work
   released prior to his break with Yogananda in 1929. Upon examination, the style
   of *The Science of Religion* is indeed much more reminiscent of Dhirananda's later
   independent publications than to anything else that Yogananda has authored.
   Dhirananda's writing does nothing to betray his Indian roots, being filled with
   references from the Bible, to Hamlet, to Bolshevism. Indeed, one might observe
   that works by New Thought authors of the time regularly employed Sanskrit with
   greater frequency than did Dhirananda's essays. However, Dhirananda's preference
   for Western terminology does little to temper the highly opaque nature of his prose
   and, like his subsequent publications, *The Science of Religion* has never enjoyed any
   notable popularity. Although it is likely that Dhirananda likewise had a significant

hand in Yogananda's initial Yogoda publications (his name appears on most editions of the pamphlet), half a decade on American soil appear to have altered Yogananda's message in a direction that left little room for philosophical abstractions.

3. Jackson 1994: 25.

4. Thomas 1930: 145.

5. Alter 2014: 66.

6. Jackson's unpublished memoir, quoted in Love 2010: 140.

7. Love 2010: 140.

8. Laycock 2013: 102.

9. From a historical point of view, Kriya Yoga, as espoused by Yogananda's lineage, displays all of the metaphysical and ritual characteristics of a medieval Indian *haṭha* yogic practice. With regards to the body of practices that came to be known as *haṭha* yoga in the modern West, this would be even more true of Yogananda's Yogoda program.

10. The first issue is concerned largely with introducing Yogananda and his work, both in India and America.

11. A corruption of the Sanskrit *yoga-da*, that is, effecting, or producing *yoga*.

12. See Singleton 2010 and Alter 2004b.

13. Alter 2005: 126.

14. Braude 2001: 151.

15. Hall 1994.

16. See Treitel 2004: 154–61.

17. Ramacharaka 1904: 11–12.

18. Ramacharaka 1904: 12.

19. *Chicago Daily Tribune* 1920.

20. X 1920.

21. Jain 2014a: 25.

22. For a full treatment of this practice, see Mallinson 2006.

23. Like most Sanskrit words, *yoni* has many meanings, the most problematic of which in this case would be that of the female sexual organ (hence, the more general meaning of "source" or "origin"). While the more anatomical sense may be implied here, even pointing to a literal practice that has been internalized over time, I believe at this stage the metaphorical meaning is a more accurate translation.

24. If one were looking to make parallels to a classical tantric *sādhana*, it seems that this stage would be akin to *nyāsa*, where a deity or deities are ritually imposed onto the practitioner's body, generally by way of mantra. The practice culminates in the practitioner's physical body, which had been ritually destroyed in the previous purificatory step of *bhūta-śuddhi*, being reconstituted as a perfected body made up entirely of *mantra* powers. It seems that, in this case, the singular *mantra* employed is "oṃ."

25. The exact distinctions regarding what exactly falls under the category of the *oṃkāra kriyās* are unclear. Dasgupta 2009: 123 actually refers to the second stage exclusively

as *thokar kriyā* and reserves the title of *oṃkāra kriyā* for the third stage where the *praṇava* sound becomes fully realized in the *brahmayoni* (the third eye).

26. On the significance of sound in the practice of *haṭha* yoga, see White 1996: 293.

27. The word "*haṃ-sa*" is seen to be a mirroring of "*so-'haṃ*," i.e. "I am That" and thus establishes an identification with the divine absolute.

28. Yogananda 1951: 374.

29. Satyananda 2004: 244.

30. Wildman 2011.

31. See Singleton 2007a. Singleton does elsewhere refer to the work of famous body-builder Maxick and his system of willed muscular flexion as a source for Yogananda's method (see Singleton 2010: 132–33), but Maxick's method, though perhaps significant in the emphasis it places on mental control of muscles, lacks the calisthenic element that distinguishes Yogananda's system. Maxick's work is, however, a more likely inspiration in the case of Yogananda's brother, bodybuilder and postural yoga pioneer Bishnu Ghosh, as will be discussed in the conclusion of this study.

32. Haddock 1921: 16–17.

33. "Ghosh Yoga & Physical Culture" 2015.

34. Yogananda 1951: 374.

35. "Yogoda Satsanga Society of India" 2015.

36. McCord 2010.

37. This entire picture is further complicated by the fact that the "swinging" exercises that form the basis of Müller's system and its ilk on the landscape of Swedish and German gymnastics were modeled on Indian club swinging. For a detailed analysis of how the colonial borrowing of physical cultural forms shaped the phenomenon of Muscular Christianity, see Alter 2004a. From this perspective, Yogananda's swinging exercises are modeled on European models of traditional Indian practices.

38. See Singleton 2010: 118, 138–39. Singleton likewise mentions that Yogendra, who would go on to be one of the main innovators of modern *āsana* practice in India, was aware of, but ultimately discounted, Müller and his body-building contemporaries as fads.

39. Singleton 2010: 140.

40. Gottschalk 1973 argues that Christian Science was at its base a religious teaching and only incidentally a healing method, while Quimbyism was a healing method and only incidentally a religious teaching. Mary Baker Eddy, Quimby's student and the founder of Christian Science, ultimately came to identify Quimbyism with Mesmerism. Associated with "occultism" as a kind of "inverted transcendence," she saw such practices as focused on the powers of the self. Eddy likewise harbored an intense distaste for spiritualism and devoted considerable attention in her foundational *Science and Health* (1875) to refuting it. She took particular pains to dissociate Christian Science from Eastern religions and Theosophy.

41. According to Albanese 2007: 195, by 1843, there were two hundred mesmerizers practicing in the Boston area alone. See also Heelas 1996.
42. Trine 1897: 18.
43. Yogananda and Dhirananda 1928: 23.
44. Yogananda and Dhirananda 1928: 23.
45. This is the subtitle of Yogananda's pamphlets.
46. Yogananda and Dhirananda 1928: 20.
47. Yogananda and Dhirananda 1928: 22.
48. Yogananda and Dhirananda 1928: 22.
49. See Singleton 2010: 56–64.
50. Yogananda and Dhirananda 1928: 23.
51. Coué 1922: 26.
52. Coué might be seen, to a large extent as replying to Payot, whose focus on the will characterizes its force as absolute but its nature as almost entirely conscious. Coué rightly observes that the efficacy of one's conscious will is significantly constrained by what one imagines to be possible. Haddock had, by this point, already mounted a similar critique in his own work, even referencing a "French writer" who states that "the Will . . . is to choose in order to act" (Haddock 1921: 17). There is no way of determining with certainty whether the mysterious French writer is in fact Payot, but this seems likely to be the case. There is likewise no way of determining whether Coué was familiar with Haddock's work (he never cites the American author). Coué would have been practicing his method contemporaneously to Haddock, but the former's publications do not arrive until the very end of his life (*My System* being published in 1923), so the lines of influence remain ambiguous. Coué differs from Haddock not so much in essence as in terminology. He defines the conscious will as a weak oppositional force to unconscious imagination, whereas Haddock views will as a general principle spanning the conscious and unconscious spectrum of human habit and volition. Yogananda, despite to a large extent replicating Haddock's language on this point, makes no mention of him.
53. Yogananda and Dhirananda 1928: 22.
54. Yogananda 1925b: 18.
55. Yogananda 1925b: 25, emphasis in original.
56. Yogoda flyer in *East-West* 4(7) (1932), emphasis in original. A version of this flyer, with slight differences in format and wording appeared in nearly every edition of the publication.
57. Singleton 2007a: 78.
58. Yogananda and Dhirananda 1928: 25.
59. Yogananda and Dhirananda 1928: 26.
60. Syman 2010: 101–2.
61. Yogananda and Dhirananda 1928: 26–27.

62. The premises of Yogananda's January 22 and January 13, 1925, lectures at the Mt. Washington center, respectively, as advertised in the *Los Angeles Times*.

63. Interestingly, this same emphasis on Christian teachings as support for the unity of religions that was so appealing to Yogananda's audiences is reported as being an alienating force for many modern seekers, who look to metaphysical and Asian-based traditions specifically to escape what they see as the oppressive influence of Christianity. See specifically Williamson 2010.

64. Yogananda 1951: 211.

65. Yogananda 1951: 212.

66. See, for instance, the account of Hilda Charlton, who received her first taste of yogic training from a man named Daya, whom she came to call the "Bogey Yogi," and his teachings regarding the Perfected Masters of Wisdom of the Great White Lodge (see Charlton 1990: 26). Yogananda was also reportedly asked if there were really masters from Lemuria living inside Mt. Shasta after some of the monks at Mt. Washington read about them in a book. To this he replied: "There have been colonists. However, no masters" (Walters 2004: 65).

67. Yogananda 1926a: 3.

68. Yogananda 1986: 231.

69. Yogananda 1926b: 4.

70. Yogananda 1926b: 4.

CHAPTER 5

1. Rinehart 1999: 95.

2. Rinehart 1999: 69.

3. Dobe 2015: 184.

4. Satyeswarananda 1991: 179.

5. As previously noted, all references to and quotes from the *Autobiography* contained in this study are taken from the 1951 edition unless otherwise specified.

6. The Indian branch of Ananda Satsanga (Kriyananda's organization) had conducted a fairly detailed study of these changes up through 1959. However, this information has since been removed from their official website. An abridged account of the changes can be found in "Changes to *Autobiography of a Yogi*" 2015.

7. Yogananda 1951: 484.

8. This, of course, suggests that the reason Yogananda has not been acknowledged as contributing to the landscape of modern postural yoga in America is because scholars assume that the SRF is an accurate representation of his teachings. However, the evidence I have cited thus far suggests that *āsana* may have been a larger aspect of practice at Yogananda's centers than I have argued even herein.

9. See, for instance, Yogananda 1951: 480.

10. See, for instance, Yogananda 1951: 222, where Yogananda states that "to fulfill one's earthly responsibilities is indeed the higher path, provided the yogi, maintaining a mental uninvolvement with egotistical desires, plays his part as a willing instrument of God."
11. Yogananda 1995: 239.
12. Satyeswarananda 1991: 183.
13. Yogananda 1951: 48.
14. Yogananda 1951: 50.
15. Yogananda 1951: 50.
16. Yogananda 1951: 54.
17. Yogananda 1951: 61.
18. Yogananda 1951: 471.
19. Yogananda 1951: 47.
20. Yogananda 1951: 140.
21. Yogananda 1951: 3.
22. Yogananda 1951: 18.
23. Yogananda 1951: 19.
24. Yogananda 1951: 20–21.
25. Yogananda 1951: 3.
26. Yogananda 1951: 86.
27. Yogananda 1951: 93.
28. Yogananda 1951: 96.
29. Yogananda 1951: 140.
30. Yogananda 1951: 154–55.
31. Yogananda 1951: 376–77.
32. Yogananda 1951: 398.
33. Yogananda 1951: 398–99.
34. Yogananda 1951: 401.
35. Yogananda 1951: 402.
36. Yogananda 1951: 410.
37. Yogananda 1951: 414.
38. Yogananda 1951: 49.
39. Yogananda 1951: 426.
40. Within Theosophical cosmologies, the astral body usually refers only to the lowest aspect of subtle embodiment. The Theosophical usage of the term is rather confusing, as Helena Blavatsky uses it interchangeably with *liṅga śarīra*, thereby also limiting the range of the original Sanskrit term. Later Theosophists, namely Annie Besant, argue that this is not in fact a proper translation and attempt to dispose with the equivalence. Since the general population of metaphysical practitioners and enthusiasts is rarely introduced to the specific subdivisions of the subtle body,

the term "astral," along with its close relative "etheric," enters the popular vocabulary as a synonym for subtle reality as a whole.

41. There are far more than sixteen known chemical elements in Yogananda's time. Likewise, the human body consists of fewer than sixteen major elements but more than sixteen once one begins to take into account its composite trace elements. It is possible that Yogananda simply thought that the number thirty-five had a nice ring to it. Thirty-five is often associated with the composite elements of Śaiva cosmologies, but there does not appear to be any further correspondence to Yogananda's system.

42. Yogananda 1951: 350.

43. Yogananda 1951: 416. There is an interesting correspondence here between Yogananda's description and Theosophical "elementals" who likewise inhabit the astral universe in Theosophical writings beginning with those of Blavatsky.

44. Yogananda 1951: 417.

45. Swedenborg's *Heaven and Hell* (1758) is the classical elaboration of his cosmology, his *Earths in the Universe* (1758) deals specifically with visions that he had of spiritually advanced being on other planets.

46. The origin of Hiranyaloka as a toponym is indeterminate. Satyeswarananda explains that it was an established notion within the tradition that disciples would always be able to locate Sri Yukteswar in "Hiranyagarva" or "Hiranyaloka" after his earthly death, specifying that, contrary to Yogananda's claims, "Hiranyaloka is not a place high up in the sky, nor is it a planet. Hiranya means 'golden,' and garva or loka means 'place.' So actually, Hiranyaloka is the area between the eyebrows where all realized souls join in oneness and union in eternal life. In fact, the inner Self, Kutastha, is the radiant Self. The radiation is golden in color, and that is why this Spot (Bindu) is called Hiranyaloka. There Sriyukteswar attained the eternal Tranquility (Brahmisthiti) or eternal Place" (Satyeswarananda 1994: 145). *Hiraṇyagarbha* is, of course, a well-known concept with multiple permutations of meaning. The term *hiraṇyagarbhaloka* appears tantalizingly in Nīlakaṇṭha's *Kriyāsāra*, a Vīraśaiva text, as designating the location to which a successful adept may advance upon meditating on certain spot on the head (line 7990). This may be simple coincidence, a concept Sri Yukteswar acquired in his vast spiritual explorations, or a hint at the deeper affiliations of the Kriya Yoga tradition.

47. This can perhaps be related to the more traditional concept that it is actually not in one's ultimate advantage to be reborn as a god in the paradisiacal *devaloka* because it is the human body that is best suited for liberation.

48. Yogananda 1951: 348.

49. Yogananda 1951: 414.

50. Yogananda 1951: 201.

51. Yogananda 1951: 426.

52. This distinction appears at the beginning of "Babaji, Yogi-Christ of Modern India" (chapter 33), in which Yogananda first fully introduces the immortal Babaji.

53. Yogananda 1951: 305.

54. Babaji's origins have since been "revealed" to the founders of the Kriya Babaji Sangh in South India (Bangalore, 1952), whom the Self Realization Fellowship has predictably tried to suppress.

55. Yogananda 1951: 310.

56. Yogananda 1951: 312.

57. Walters 2004: 347.

58. See White 2009: 168 and chapter 1 in this book.

EPILOGUE

1. This range of years is the best approximation I could arrive at. The exact program that featured this segment is unknown. A number of such clips were in possession of Choudhury's headquarters, collected by his senior teachers, and were made available on the Internet (the video in my possession was retrieved in March 2010) until they were inexplicably taken down, presumably due to copyright issues.

2. Lorr 2012: 287n29.

3. Martin 2011.

4. Lorr 2012: 140.

5. Lorr 2012: 150.

6. The following account draws on Choudhury 2007, Lorr 2012, information disseminated by the Bishnu Ghosh Lineage Project, and anecdotal accounts passed around by Choudhury's senior teachers and acolytes.

7. Choudhury 2007: 28.

8. Lorr 2012: 25. Apparently, Ghosh had previously declared that a heart attack would be the most pleasant mode of death.

9. The introduction of the heated room definitely happened. No evidence of Japanese scientific articles or of Choudhury's encounter with Nixon has ever been found.

10. Yoga Journal and Yoga Alliance's 2016 "Yoga in America" study found that 36 million Americans practice some form of yoga and that they annually spend roughly $16 billion to do so. See "Yoga in America Study" 2016.

11. Choudhury 2007: 32.

12. For a detailed account, see Fish 2006.

13. Susman 2005: 274.

14. Choudhury 2014.

15. Lorr 2012: 153–55.

16. Walters 2004: 189. For a "fanfiction-esque" account of Yogananda's life as William the Conqueror and his connection to Kriyananda as his then-son, Henry I, see Kairavi 2010.

17. Bender 2010: 185.

18. Lindsay 1996: 357–58.

19. This term originates from theoretical physics. However, David White (2014) has argued that it can also be used to describe the projects of such yogic sources as the *Yoga Sūtras*.

20. Alter 2006a: 767.

21. Although the characters of *Heroes* for the most part do not actively seek to cultivate these superpowers, the series nevertheless suggests that such abilities may present an evolutionary advance that points to the superhuman potential of every human being, in line with the theories presented by Vivekananda and Yogananda.

22. For more on Tesla's interest in intersections between science and the occult, see Pokazanyeva 2016: 335–39.

23. This version of the character debuted in *Doctor Strange* #177 (1969), where a plot point necessitated that Strange take on a different form. It is sometimes known as the Blue Mage or Necromancer costume.

24. For the implications of religious *bricolage* and appropriation, see Altglas 2014.

25. Bender 2010: 112.

26. Kadetsky 2004: 82–83.

27. See Malhotra 2001: 89–99.

Bibliography

Abhedananda, Swami. 1902. *How to Be a Yogi*. New York: The Vedanta Society.

Adams, Barbara. 1935. "Yogi Pretends 'Hindu Lore' Is Key to All Ills." *Chicago Daily Tribune*, February 7.

Albanese, Catherine L. 1999. "The Subtle Energies of Spirit: Explorations in Metaphysical and New Age Spirituality." *Journal of the American Academy of Religion* 67 (2): 305–25.

Albanese, Catherine L. 2005. "Sacred (and Secular) Self-Fashioning: Esalen and the American Transformation of Yoga." In *On the Edge of the Future: Esalen and the Evolution of American Culture*, edited by Jeffrey J. Kripal and Glen W. Shuck, 45–79. Bloomington: Indiana University Press.

Albanese, Catherine L. 2007. *A Republic of Mind and Spirit: A Cultural History of American Metaphysical Religion*. New Haven: Yale University Press.

Alexander, Mrs. Gross. 1912. "American Women Going after Heathen Gods." *Methodist Quarterly Review* 61 (July): 495–512.

Alter, Joseph S. 1994. "Somatic Nationalism: Indian Wrestling and Militant Hinduism." *Modern Asian Studies* 28 (3): 557–88.

Alter, Joseph S. 2000. *Gandhi's Body: Sex, Diet, and the Politics of Nationalism*. Philadelphia: University of Pennsylvania Press.

Alter, Joseph S. 2004a. "Indian Clubs and Colonialism: Hindu Masculinity and Muscular Christianity." *Comparative Studies in Society and History* 46 (3): 497–534.

Alter, Joseph S. 2004b. *Yoga in Modern India: The Body between Science and Philosophy*. Princeton: Princeton University Press.

Alter, Joseph S. 2005. "Modern Medical Yoga: Struggling with a History of Magic, Alchemy and Sex." *Asian Medicine* 1: 119–46.

Alter, Joseph S. 2006a. "Yoga and Fetishism: Reflections on Marxist Social Theory." *Journal of the Royal Anthropological Institute* 12: 763–83.

Alter, Joseph S. 2006b. "Yoga at the Fin de Siècle: Muscular Christianity with a 'Hindu' Twist." *International Journal of the History of Sport* 23 (5): 759–76.

Alter, Joseph S. 2011a. *Moral Materialism: Sex and Masculinity in Modern India*. New Delhi: Penguin Books.

Alter, Joseph S. 2011b. "Yoga, Modernity and the Middle-Class: Locating the Body in a World of Desire." In *A Companion to the Anthropology of India*, edited by Isabelle Clark-Decès, 154–68. Hoboken, NJ: Wiley-Blackwell.

Alter, Joseph S. 2014. "Shri Yogendra: Magic, Modernity and the Burden of the Middle-Class Yogi." In *Gurus of Modern Yoga*, edited by Mark Singleton and Ellen Goldberg, 60–82. New York: Oxford University Press.

Altglas, Véronique. 2014. *From Yoga to Kabbalah: Religious Exoticism and the Logics of Bricolage*. New York: Oxford University Press.

Altman, Michael J. 2013. "Imagining Hindus: India and Religion in Nineteenth Century America." PhD diss., Emory University.

Angel, Leonard. 1994. *Enlightenment East and West*. Albany: State University of New York Press.

Arnold, Edwin. 1879. *Light of Asia; or, the Great Renunciation*. New York: A. L. Burt.

Atkinson, William Walker. 1906. *Thought Vibration or the Law of Attraction in the Thought World*. Chicago: The Library Shelf.

Atulananda, Swami. 1938. *With the Swamis in America*. Mayavati: Advaita Ashrama.

Asprem, Egil. 2014. *The Problem of Disenchantment: Scientific Naturalism and Esoteric Discourse, 1900–1939*. Leiden: Brill.

Bald, Vivek. 2013. *Bengali Harlem and the Lost Histories of South Asian America*. Cambridge, MA: Harvard University Press.

Beckerlegge, Gwilym. 2013. "Swami Vivekananda (1863–1902) 150 Years on: Critical Studies of an Influential Hindu Guru." *Religion Compass* 7 (10): 444–53.

Bednarowski, Mary Farrell. 1980. "Outside the Mainstream: Women's Religion and Women Religious Leaders in Nineteenth-Century America." *Journal of the American Academy of Religion* 48 (2): 207–31.

Bender, Courtney. 2010. *The New Metaphysicals: Spirituality and the American Religious Imagination*. Chicago: University of Chicago Press.

Bernard, Theos. 1950. *Hatha Yoga: The Report of a Personal Experience*. London: Rider.

Bernier, François. 1976. *Travels in the Mogul Empire, A.D. 1656–1668*. Translated by Brock Irving and Archibald Constable. Lahore: al-Biruni.

Biernacki, Loriliai. 2007. *The Renowned Goddess of Desire: Women, Sex and Speech in Tantra*. New York: Oxford University Press.

Blavatsky, H. P. 1877. *Isis Unveiled: A Master-Key to the Mysteries of Ancient and Modern Science and Theology*. New York: J. W. Bouton.

Blavatsky, H. P. 1954. *Collected Writings*. Vol. 6. Edited by Boris De Zirkoff. Wheaton, IL: Theosophical Publishing House.

Blavatsky, H. P. 1966. *Collected Writings*. Vol. 1. Edited by Boris De Zirkoff. Wheaton, IL: Theosophical Publishing House.

Blavatsky, H. P. 1969. *Collected Writings*. Vol. 4. Edited by Boris De Zirkoff. Wheaton, IL: Theosophical Publishing House.

Blavatsky, H. P. 1980. *Collected Writings*. Vol. 12. Edited by Boris De Zirkoff. Wheaton, IL: Theosophical Publishing House.

Bouillier, Véronique. 1989. "Des prêtres du pouvoir: Les yogī et la fonction royale." In *Prêtrise, pouvoirs et autorité en Himalaya*, edited by Véronique Bouillier and Gerard Toffin, 193–214. Paris: Editions de l'Ecole des Hautes Études en Sciences Sociales.

Braden, Charles Samuel. 1963. *Spirits in Rebellion: The Rise and Development of New Thought*. Dallas, TX: Southern Methodist University Press.

Brain, Robert Michael. 2013. "Materialising the Medium: Ectoplasm and the Quest for Supranormal Biology in Fin-de-Siècle Science and Art." In *Vibratory Modernism*, edited by Anthony Enns and Shelley Trower, 115–44. New York: Palgrave Macmillan.

Braude, Ann. 2001. *Radical Spirits: Spiritualism and Women's Rights in Nineteenth-Century America*. Bloomington: Indiana University Press.

Breckenridge, Carol Appadurai, and Peter Van der Veer, eds. 1993. *Orientalism and the Postcolonial Predicament: Perspectives on South Asia*. Philadelphia: University of Pennsylvania Press.

Brekke, Torkel. 2002. *Makers of Modern Indian Religion in the Late Nineteenth Century*. Oxford: Oxford University Press.

Brown, C. Mackenzie. 2007. "The Western Roots of Avataric Evolutionism in Colonial India." *Zygon* 42 (2): 423–48.

Brunner, Hélène. 1975. "Le Sādhaka, personnage oublié du śivaïsme du sud." *Journal Asiatique* 263: 411–43.

Brunton, Paul. 1935. *A Search in Secret India*. New York: E. P. Dutton.

Bühnemann, Gudrun. 2007. *Eighty-Four Āsanas in Yoga: A Survey of Traditions, with Illustrations*. New Delhi: D. K. Printworld.

Burke, Marie Louise. 1958. *Swami Vivekananda in America: New Discoveries*. Calcutta: Advaita Ashrama.

Cameron, Kenneth Walter. 1954. *Indian Superstition*. Hanover: Friends of the Dartmouth Library.

Campbell, Bruce F. 1980. *Ancient Wisdom Revived: A History of the Theosophical Movement*. Berkeley: University of California Press.

Cantor, G. N., and M. J. S. Hodge, eds. 1981. *Conceptions of Ether: Studies in the History of Ether Theories, 1740–1900*. Cambridge: Cambridge University Press.

Carroll, Bret E. 1997. *Spiritualism in Antebellum America*. Bloomington: Indiana University Press.

"Changes to Autobiography of a Yogi." 2015. *Yogananda for the World*. http://www.yoganandafortheworld.com/changes-to-autobiography-of-a-yogi/.

Charlton, Hilda. 1990. *Hell-Bent for Heaven: The Autobiography of Hilda Charlton*. Woodstock, NY: Golden Quest.

Chicago Daily Tribune. 1902. "Home Course in New Thought." March 19.

Chicago Daily Tribune. 1911. "Raja Yogi Cult Gets into Court: Witness Testifies of Weird Hindu Rites Practiced by Late Mrs. Ole Bull." May 24.

Choudhury, Bikram. 2007. *Bikram Yoga: The Guru Behind Hot Yoga Shows the Way to Radiant Health and Personal Fulfillment*. New York: Harper Collins Publishers.

Choudhury, Bikram. 2014. "Press Release." http://www.bikramyoga.com.

Christy, Arthur. 1932. *The Orient in American Transcendentalism: A Study of Emerson, Thoreau, and Alcott*. New York: Columbia University Press.

Cohen, Jeffrey Jerome, ed. 1996. *Monster Theory: Reading Culture*. Minneapolis: University of Minnesota Press.

Copley, Antony, ed. 2000. *Gurus and Their Followers: New Religious Reform Movements in Colonial India*. New Delhi: Oxford University Press.

Coué, Émile. 1922. *Self Mastery through Conscious Autosuggestion*. New York: Malkan.

Crabtree, Adam. 1993. *From Mesmer to Freud: Magnetic Sleep and the Roots of Psychological Healing*. New Haven: Yale University Press.

Cullen, Frank, Florence Hackman, and Donald McNeilly, eds. 2007. "Jovedah." *Vaudeville Old & New: An Encyclopedia of Variety Performers in America*, 580. New York: Routledge.

Daggett, Mabel Potter. 1911. "The Heathen Invasion." *Hampton-Columbian Magazine* 27 (October): 399–411.

Dare, M. Paul. 1940. *Indian Underworld: A First-Hand Account of Hindu Saints, Sorcerers, and Superstitions*. New York: E. P. Dutton.

Dasgupta, Sailendra Bejoy. 2006. *Paramhansa Swami Yogananda: Life Portrait and Reminiscences*. Translated by Yoga Niketan. Lincoln: iUniverse.

Dasgupta, Sailendra Bejoy. 2009. *Kriya Yoga*. Translated by Yoga Niketan. Lincoln: iUniverse.

Davis, Roy Eugene. 2006. *Paramahansa Yogananda as I Knew Him: Experiences, Observations, and Reflections of a Disciple*. New Delhi: Full Circle Publishers.

Dazey, Wade. 2005. "Yoga in America: Some Reflections from the Heartland." In *Theory and Practice of Yoga: Essays in Honour of James Gerald Larson*, edited by Knut A. Jacobsen, 409–24. Boston: Brill.

Dehejia, Vidya. 1986. *Yoginī Cult and Temples: A Tantric Tradition*. New Delhi: National Museum.

De Michelis, Elizabeth. 2004. *A History of Modern Yoga: Patañjali and Western Esoterism*. London: Continuum.

Deslippe, Philip. 2014. "The Hindu in Hoodoo: Fake Yogis, Pseudo-Swamis, and the Manufacture of African American Folk Magic." *Amerasia Journal* 40 (1): 34–56.

Deslippe, Philip. 2015. "The Lost Early History of Yoga in America." California Polytechnic State University, San Luis Obispo, May 19.

Dhirananda, Swami. 1926a. *Glimpses of Light: A Collection of Excerpts from Sermons on Oriental and Occidental Philosophies and Religions*. Los Angeles: Aetna.

Dhirananda, Swami. 1926b. *Philosophic Insight (A Message in Essays)*. Los Angeles: Sat-Sanga, Mt. Washington Educational Center.

Diamond, Debra, ed. 2013. *Yoga: The Art of Transformation*. Washington, DC: Smithsonian Institution.

Dillon, Jane Robinson. 1998. "The Social Significance of a Western Belief in Reincarnation: A Qualitative Study of the Self-Realization Fellowship." PhD diss., University of California, San Diego.

Dobe, Timothy. 2015. *Hindu Christian Faqir: Modern Monks, Global Christianity, and Indian Sainthood*. New York: Oxford University Press.

Doniger O'Flaherty, Wendy. 1981. *Śiva, the Erotic Ascetic*. New York: Oxford University Press.

Duquette, Jonathan, and K. Ramasubramanian. 2010. "Is Space Created?: Reflections on Śaṇkara's Philosophy and Philosophy of Physics." *Philosophy East and West* 60 (4): 517–33.

Einstein, Albert. 1920. "Aether and the Theory of Relativity." University of Leyden, Germany. http://www.aetherometry.com/Electronic_Publications/Science/einstein_aether_and_relativity.php.

Ellwood, Robert S. 1979. *Alternative Altars: Unconventional and Eastern Spirituality in America*. Chicago: University of Chicago Press.

Ellwood, Robert S. 1983. "The American Theosophical Synthesis." In *The Occult in America: New Historical Perspectives*, edited by Howard Kerr and Charles L. Crow, 111–34. Urbana: University of Illinois Press.

Ernst, Carl W. 2003. "The Islamization of Yoga in the 'Amrtakunda' Translations." *Journal of the Royal Asiatic Society* 13 (2): 199–226.

Ernst, Carl W. 2005. "Situating Sufism and Yoga." *Journal of the Royal Asiatic Society* 15 (1): 15–43.

Esdaile, James. 1846. *Mesmerism in India and Its Practical Application in Surgery and Medicine*. London: Longman, Brown, Green, and Longmans.

Evans, Warren Felt. 1886. *Esoteric Christianity and Mental Therapeutics*. Boston: H. H. Carter and Karrick.

Farquhar, J[ohn] N[icol]. 1967. *Modern Religious Movements in India*. Delhi: Munshiran Manoharlal.

Fish, Allison. 2006. "The Commodification and Exchange of Knowledge in the Case of Transnational Commercial Yoga." *International Journal of Cultural Property* 13: 189–206.

Flood, Gavin. 2006. *The Tantric Body: The Secret Tradition of Hindu Religion*. London: I. B. Tauris.

Forsthoefel, Thomas A., and Cynthia Ann Humes, eds. 2005. *Gurus in America*. Albany: State University of New York Press.

Francavigalia, Richard V. 2011. *Go East, Young Man: Imagining the American West as the Orient*. Logan: Utah State University Press.

Fueurstein, Georg. 1991. *Holy Madness: The Shock Tactics and Radical Teachings of Crazy-Wise Adepts, Holy Fools, and Rascal Gurus*. New York: Paragon House.

Fuller, Robert C. 1982. *Mesmerism and the American Cure of Souls.* Philadelphia: University of Pennsylvania Press.

Gandhi, Shreena Niketa Divyakant. 2009. "Translating, Practicing and Commodifying Yoga in the U.S." PhD diss., University of Florida.

Garland-Thomson, Rosemarie, ed. 1996. *Freakery: Cultural Spectacles of the Extraordinary Body.* New York: New York University Press.

Ghosh, Sananda Lal. 1980. *Mejda: The Family and Early Life of Paramahansa Yogananda.* Los Angeles: Self-Realization Fellowship.

"Ghosh Yoga & Physical Culture." 2015. http://www.ghoshyoga.com.

Gleig, Ann, and Lola Williamson, eds. 2014. *Homegrown Gurus: From Hinduism in America to American Hinduism.* Albany: State University of New York Press.

Goldberg, Philip. 2010. *American Veda: From Emerson and the Beatles to Yoga and Meditation: How Indian Spirituality Changed the West.* New York: Harmony Books.

Gold, Daniel. 1988. *Comprehending the Guru: Toward a Grammar of Religious Perception.* Atlanta, GA: Scholars Press.

Gottschalk, Stephen. 1973. *The Emergence of Christian Science in American Religious Life.* Berkeley: University of California Press.

Govindan, Marshall. 1991. *Babaji and the 18 Siddha Kriya Yoga Tradition.* Montreal: Kriya Yoga Publication.

Gupta, Sanjukta. 1972. *Lakṣmī Tantra: A Pāñcarātra Text.* Leiden: Brill.

Gutierrez, Cathy. 2009. *Plato's Ghost: Spiritualism in the American Renaissance.* New York: Oxford University Press.

Hackett, Paul G. 2012. *Theos Bernard, the White Lama: Tibet, Yoga, and American Religious Life.* New York: Columbia University Press.

Haddock, Franck Channing. 1921. *Power of Will: A Practical Companion Book for Unfoldment of the Powers of Mind.* Meriden, CT: Pelton.

Hall, Donald E. 1994. *Muscular Christianity: Embodying the Victorian Age.* New York: Cambridge University Press.

Hanegraaff, Wouter J. 1996. *New Age Religion and Western Culture: Esotericism in the Mirror of Secular Thought.* Leiden: Brill.

Harper, Marvin Henry. 1972. *Gurus, Swamis, and Avataras: Spiritual Masters and Their American Disciples.* Philadelphia: Westminster Press.

Hatley, Shaman. 2007. "Mapping the Esoteric Body in the Islamic Yoga of Bengal." *History of Religions* 46 (4): 351–68.

Hauser, Beatrix, ed. 2013. *Yoga Traveling: Bodily Practice in Transcultural Perspective.* New York: Springer.

Heehs, Peter. 2003. "Shades of Orientalism: Paradoxes and Problems in Indian Historiography." *History and Theory* 42 (2): 169–95.

Heehs, Peter. 2008. *The Lives of Sri Aurobindo.* New York: Columbia University Press.

Heelas, Paul. 1996. *The New Age Movement: The Celebration of the Self and the Sacralization of Modernity.* Oxford: Blackwell.

Holdrege, Barbara A. 1996. *Veda and Torah: Transcending the Textuality of Scripture.* Albany: State University of New York Press.

Horowitz, Mitch. 2009. *Occult America: The Secret History of How Mysticism Shaped Our Nation.* New York: Bantam Books.

Howard, David H. 1974. "Yesterday's Evangelist from India." *A. K. Mozumdar.* http://www.mozumdar.org/yesterdaysevangelist.html.

Hutchinson, Brian. 1992. "The Divine-Human Figure in the Transmission of Religious Tradition." In *A Sacred Thread: Modern Transmission of Hindu Traditions in India and Abroad,* edited by Raymond Brady Williams, 92–126. New York: Columbia University Press.

Isaacs, Harold R. 1958. *Images of Asia: American Views of China and India.* New York: Capricorn Books.

Isherwood, Christopher. 1965. *Ramakrishna and His Disciples.* New York: Simon and Schuster.

Iwamura, Jane Naomi. 2011. *Virtual Orientalism: Asian Religions and American Popular Culture.* New York: Oxford University Press.

Jackson, Carl T. 1981. *The Oriental Religions and American Thought: Nineteenth-Century Explorations.* Westport, CT: Greenwood Press.

Jackson, Carl T. 1994. *Vedanta for the West: The Ramakrishna Movement in the United States.* Bloomington: Indiana University Press.

Jacobsen, Knut A., ed. 2011. *Yoga Powers: Extraordinary Capacities Attained through Meditation and Concentration.* Leiden: Brill.

Jain, Andrea R. 2014a. *Selling Yoga: From Counterculture to Pop Culture.* New York: Oxford University Press.

Jain, Andrea R. 2014b. "Who Is to Say Modern Yoga Practitioners Have It All Wrong? On Hindu Origins and Yogaphobia." *Journal of the American Academy of Religion* 82 (2): 427–71.

Johnson, K. Paul. 1994. *The Masters Revealed: Madame Blavatsky and the Myth of the Great White Lodge.* Albany: State University of New York Press.

Jung-Stilling, Johan Heinrich, and Samuel Jackson. 1844. *The Autobiography of Heinrich Stilling, Late Aulic Counsellor to the Grand Duke of Baden, &c., &c., &c.* Translated by W. H. E. Schwartz. New York: Harper and Brothers.

Kadetsky, Elizabeth. 2004. *First There Is a Mountain: A Yoga Romance.* Boston: Little, Brown.

Kairavi, Catherine. 2010. *Two Souls, Four Lives: The Lives and Former Lives of Paramhansa Yogananda and His Disciple, Swami Kriyananda.* Nevada City, CA: Crystal Clarity.

Keegan, Paul. 2012. "Yogis Behaving Badly." *Business 2.0,* September.

Killingly, D. H. 1990. "Yoga-Sutra IV, 2–3 and Vivekananda's Interpretation of Evolution." *Journal of Indian Philosophy* 18 (2): 151–79.

King, Richard. 1999. *Orientalism and Religion: Postcolonial Theory, India and "The Mystic East."* London: Routledge.

Knowles, Christopher. 2007. *Our Gods Wear Spandex: The Secret History of Comic Book Heroes*. San Francisco, CA: Weiser Books.

Kopf, David. 1969. *British Orientalism and the Bengal Renaissance: The Dynamics of Indian Modernization, 1773–1835*. Berkeley: University of California Press.

Kopf, David. 1979. *The Brahmo Samaj and the Shaping of the Modern Indian Mind*. Princeton: Princeton University Press.

Kostro, Ludwik. 2000. *Einstein and the Ether*. Montreal: Apeiron.

Kramer, Paul A. 2011. "The Importance of Being Turbaned." *Antioch Review* 69 (2): 208–21.

Kripal, Jeffrey J. 2010. *Authors of the Impossible: The Paranormal and the Sacred*. Chicago: University of Chicago Press.

Kripal, Jeffrey J. 2011. *Mutants and Mystics: Science Fiction, Superhero Comics, and the Paranormal*. Chicago: University of Chicago Press.

Kriyananda, Swami. 2010. *Rescuing Yogananda*. Nevada City, CA: Crystal Clarity Publishers.

Kriyananda, Swami. 2011. *Paramhansa Yogananda: A Biography, with Personal Reflections and Reminiscences*. Nevada City, CA: Crystal Clarity Publishers.

Lal, Vinay, and Leela Prasad. 1999. "Establishing Roots, Engendering Awareness: A Political History of Asian Indians in the United States." In *Live like the Banyan Tree: Images of the Indian American Experience*, 42–28. Philadelphia: Balch Institute for Ethnic Studies.

Lamont, Peter. 2004. *The Rise of the Indian Rope Trick: The Biography of a Legend*. London: Little, Brown.

Larson, Gerald James, and Ram Shankar Bhattacharya, eds. 2008. *Yoga: India's Philosophy of Meditation*. Delhi: Motilal Banarsidass Publishers.

Laycock, Joseph. 2013. "Yoga for the New Woman and the New Man: The Role of Pierre Bernard and Blanche DeVriesin the Creation of Modern Postural Yoga." *Religion and American Culture: A Journal of Interpretation* 23 (1): 101–36.

Lee, Robert G. 1999. *Orientals: Asian Americans in Popular Culture*. Philadelphia: Temple University Press.

Leeman, Lisa, and Paola di Florio. 2014. *Awake: The Life of Yogananda*. DVD. New York: Alive Mind Cinema.

Lindsay, Cecile, and Rosemarie Garland-Thomson. 1996. "Body Building: A Postmodern Freak Show." In *Freakery: Cultural Spectacles of the Extraordinary Body*, 356–67. New York: New York University Press.

Lorenzen, David N., and Adrián Muñoz, eds. 2011. *Yogi Heroes and Poets: Histories and Legends of the Naths*. Albany: State University of New York Press.

Lorr, Benjamin. 2012. *Hell-Bent: Obsession, Pain, and the Search for Something like Transcendence in Bikram Yoga*. London: Bloomsbury.

Los Angeles Times. 1910. "Massaging Too Much for Her: Woman Causes Hindu Hypnotist's Downfall." May 14.

Los Angeles Times. 1919. "Was the Club Yogi Colony?: Strange Rites of Peculiar People at Nyack, N.Y." November 28.

Los Angeles Times. 1923. "Make Yourself Venus: All That's Necessary Is Will Power; Coue Is Fairly Out-Coued by New Yogi Who Is Coming." March 4.

Los Angeles Times. 1926. "Yogi Philosophy Blamed by Wife in Divorce Plea." January 20.

Los Angeles Times. 1928. "Swami Returns from East: Mt. Washington Cult Teacher Taken from Train at San Bernardino." January 15.

Los Angeles Times. 1935a. "Swami Row to Be Aired: Trial of Suit Involving India Religious Leaders Scheduled Today." August 21.

Los Angeles Times. 1935b. "Swami Assails Swami in Litigation over Note." August 23.

Los Angeles Times. 1939. "Swami Sued for $500,000: Action Charges Girls Living at Headquarters of Religious Leader." October 24.

Los Angeles Times. 1940a. "Swami Fights $500,000 Aide's Demand in Court." December 4.

Los Angeles Times. 1940b. "Swami's Share Profits Pledge Told at Trial." December 5.

Love, Robert. 2010. *The Great Oom: The Improbable Birth of Yoga in America*. New York: Viking.

Malhotra, Ashok Kumar. 2001. *An Introduction to Yoga Philosophy: An Annotated Translation of the Yoga Sutras*. Burlington, VT: Ashgate.

Mallinson, James. 2006. *The Khecarīvidyā of Ādinātha: A Critical and Annotated Translation of an Early Text of Haṭhayoga*. London: Routledge.

Martin, Clancy. 2011. "The Overheated, Oversexed Cult of Bikram Choudhury." *Details*. February 1. http://www.details.com/culture-trends/critical-eye/201102/yoga-guru-bikram-choudhury.

Mayo, Katherine. 1927. *Mother India*. New York: Harcourt, Brace.

McCord, Gyandev. 2010. "Yogananda's Views on Hatha Yoga." *The Expanding Light*. September 10. http://www.expandinglight.org/free/yoga-teacher/articles/gyandev/Yoganandas-Views-on-Hatha-Yoga.php.

McKean, Lise. 1996. *Divine Enterprise: Gurus and the Hindu Nationalist Movement*. Chicago: University of Chicago Press.

Melton, J. Gordon. 1989. "The Attitude of Americans toward Hinduism from 1883 to 1893 with Special Reference to the International Society for Krishna Consciousness." In *Krishna Consciousness in the West*, edited by David G. Bromley and Larry D. Shinn, 79–101. Lewisburg, PA: Bucknell University Press.

Meyer, Donald. 1965. *The Positive Thinkers: A Study of the American Quest for Health, Wealth and Personal Power from Mary Baker Eddy to Norman Vincent Peale*. New York: Doubleday.

Miami Daily News. 1928a. "Quigg Resents Yogi's Effort at Hypnotizing." February 2.

Miami Daily News. 1928b. "Dozen Witnesses Flay Swami." February 8.

Milutis, Joe. 2006. *Ether: The Nothing That Connects Everything*. Minneapolis: University of Minnesota Press.

Moloney, Deirdre M. 2012. *National Insecurities: Immigrants and U.S. Deportation Policy since 1882*. Chapel Hill: University of North Carolina Press.

Moore, Laurence R. 1977. *In Search of White Crows: Spiritualism, Parapsychology, and American Culture*. New York: Oxford University Press.

Nance, Susan. 2009. *How the Arabian Nights Inspired the American Dream, 1790–1935*. Chapel Hill: University of North Carolina Press.

Narayan, Kirin. 1993. "Refractions of the Field at Home: American Representations of Hindu Holy Men in the 19th and 20th Centuries." *Cultural Anthropology* 8 (4): 476–509.

Newcombe, Suzanne. 2009. "The Development of Modern Yoga: A Survey of the Field." *The Religion Compass* 3 (6): 986–1002.

New Pilgrimages of the Spirit: Proceedings and Papers of the Pilgrim Tercentenary Meeting of the International Congress of Free Christian and Other Religious Liberals, Held at Boston and Plymouth, U.S.A., October 3–7, 1920. 1921. Boston: Beacon Press.

New York Times. 1909. "Hold 'Yogi' Garnett for Duping Women: Fortune Teller Wanted Here for Mining Stock Swindle Caught After Years' Search." October 19.

New York Times. 1927. "Fakir Buried for Hours, Beats Houdini Time." January 21.

New York Times. 1928. "Swami's Lectures to Women Face Ban as Miami Official Foresees Violence." February 4.

Noakes, Richard. 2007. "Cromwell Varley FRS, Electrical Discharge and Victorian Spiritualism." *Notes and Record of the Royal Society of London* 61 (1): 5–21.

Noakes, Richard. 2008. "The 'World of the Infinitely Little': Connecting Physical and Psychical Realities Circa 1900." *Studies in History and Philosophy of Science* 39: 323–34.

Olcott, Henry Steel. 1875. *People from the Other World*. Hartford: American Publishing Company.

Oman, John Campbell. 1889. *Indian Life: Religious and Social*. London: T. Fisher Unwin.

Oman, John Campbell. 1903. *The Mystics, Ascetics, and Saints of India: A Study of Sadhuism, with an Account of Yogis, Bairagis, and Other Strange Hindu Sectarians*. London: T. Fisher Unwin.

Owen, Alex. 1990. *The Darkened Room: Women, Power, and Spiritualism in Late Victorian England*. Philadelphia: University of Pennsylvania Press.

Owen, Alex. 2007. *The Place of Enchantment: British Occultism and the Culture of the Modern*. Chicago: University of Chicago Press.

"Paramahansa Yogananda's Complete Mortuary Report." 1952. Forest Lawn Memorial-Park, Harry T. Rowe, Mortuary Director.

Parker, Gail Thain. 1973. *Mind Cure in New England: From the Civil War to World War I*. Hanover: University Press of New England.

Payot, Jules. 1909. *The Education of the Will: The Theory and Practise of Self-Culture*. New York: Funk and Wagnalls.

Pinch, William R. 2006. *Warrior Ascetics and Indian Empires*. New York: Cambridge University Press.

Poe, Edgar Allan. 1966. *Complete Stories and Poems of Edgar Allan Poe*. Garden City, NY: Doubleday.

Pokazanyeva, Anna. 2016. "Mind within Matter: Science, the Occult, and the (Meta) physics of Ether and Akasha." *Zygon* 51 (2): 318–46.

Pollock, Sheldon. 1993. "Deep Orientalism? Notes on Sanskrit and Power beyond the Raj." In *Orientalism and the Post-Colonial Predicament: Perspectives on South Asia*, edited by Carol A. Breckenridge and Van der Veer, 76–133. Philadelphia: University of Pennsylvania Press.

Prasada, Rama. 1894. *The Science of Breath and the Philosophy of the Tattvas*. London: Theosophical Publishing Society.

Prothero, Stephen. 2004. "Hinduphobia and Hinduphilia in U.S. Culture." In *The Stranger's Religion: Fascination and Fear*, 13–37. Notre Dame: University of Notre Dame Press.

Radice, William. 1998. *Swami Vivekananda and the Modernization of Hinduism*. Delhi: Oxford University Press.

Raia, Courtenay Grean. 2007. "From Ether Theory to Ether Theology: Oliver Lodge and the Physics of Immortality." *Journal of the History of Behavioral Sciences* 43 (1): 19–43.

Ramacharaka, Yogi. 1903. *The Hindu-Yogi Science of Breath: A Complete Manual of the Oriental Breathing Philosophy of Physical, Mental, Psychic and Spiritual Development*. Chicago: Yogi Publication Society.

Ramacharaka, Yogi. 1904. *Hatha Yoga; or, the Yogi Philosophy of Physical Well-Being*. Chicago: Yogi Publication Society.

Ramacharaka, Yogi. 1931. *Fourteen Lessons in Yogi Philosophy and Oriental Occultism*. Chicago: Yogi Publication Society.

Rastelli, Marion. 2000. "The Religious Practice of the Sādhaka According to the Jayākhyasaṃhitā." *Indo-Iranian Journal* 43: 219–95.

Reed, Elizabeth A. 1914. *Hinduism in Europe and America*. New York: G. P. Putnam's Sons.

Rinehart, Robin. 1999. *One Lifetime, Many Lives: The Experience of Modern Hindu Hagiography*. Atlanta, GA: Scholars Press.

Rocklin, Alexander. 2016. "'A Hindu Is White Although He Is Black': Hindu Alterity and the Performativity of Religion and Race between the United States and the Caribbean." *Comparative Studies in Society and History* 58 (1): 181–210.

Rose, H. A. 1916. "Magic (Indian)." In *Encyclopoedia of Religion and Ethics*, edited by James Hastings. New York: Charles Scribner's Sons.

Rosser, Brenda Lewis. 1991. *Treasures Against Time: Paramahansa Yogananda with Doctor and Mrs. Lewis*. Borrego Springs, CA: Borrego Publications.

Said, Edward W. 1978. *Orientalism*. New York: Pantheon Books.

Sarbacker, Stuart Ray. 2005. *Samādhi: The Numinous and Cessative in Indo-Tibetan Yoga*. Albany: State University of New York Press.

Sarbacker, Stuart Ray. 2011. "Power and Meaning in the Yogasūtra of Patañjali." In *Yoga Powers: Extraordinary Capacities Attained Through Meditation and Concentration*, edited by Knut A. Jacobsen, 195–222. Leiden: Brill.

Satter, Beryl. 1999. *Each Mind a Kingdom: American Women, Sexual Purity, and the New Thought Movement, 1875–1920*. Berkeley: University of California Press.

Satyananda, Swami. 2004. *A Collection of Biographies of 4 Kriya Yoga Gurus*. Translated by Yoga Niketan. Lincoln: iUniverse.

Satyeswarananda Giri, Swami. 1983. *Lahiri Mahasay: The Father of Kriya Yoga*. San Diego, CA: Swami Satyeswarananda Giri.

Satyeswarananda Giri, Swami. 1984. *Babaji: The Divine Himalayan Yogi*. San Diego, CA: Swami Satyeswarananda Giri.

Satyeswarananda Giri, Swami. 1985. *Kebalananda and Sriyukteswar: Biographies*. San Diego, CA: Swami Satyeswarananda Giri.

Satyeswarananda Giri, Swami. 1991. *Kriya: Finding the True Path*. San Diego, CA: Sanskrit Classics.

Satyeswarananda Giri, Swami. 1994. *Sriyukteswar: A Biography*. San Diego, CA: Sanskrit Classics.

Schmidt, Leigh Eric. 2010. *Heaven's Bride: The Unprintable Life of Ida C. Craddock, American Mystic, Scholar, Sexologist, Martyr, and Madwoman*. New York: Basic Books.

Schrödinger, Erwin. 1956. *Mind and Matter*. Cambridge: Cambridge University Press.

Schrödinger, Erwin. 1964. *My View of the World*. Cambridge: Cambridge University Press.

Seager, Richard Hughes. 1993. *The Dawn of Religious Pluralism: Voices from the World's Parliament of Religions 1893*. La Salle, IL: Open Court.

Seager, Richard Hughes. 1995. *The World's Parliament of Religions: The East/West Encounter, Chicago, 1893*. Bloomington: Indiana University Press.

Shaw, Miranda. 1995. *Passionate Enlightenment: Women in Tantric Buddhism*. Princeton: Princeton University Press.

Shontell, Alyson. 2013. "The Last Gift Steve Jobs Gave to Family and Friends Was a Book about Self Realization." *Business Insider*, September 11. http://www.businessinsider.com/steve-jobs-gave-yoganandas-book-as-a-gift-at-his-memorial-2013-9.

Siegel, Lee. 1991. *Net of Magic: Wonders and Deceptions in India*. Chicago: University of Chicago Press.

Siegel, Lee. 2014. *Trance-Migrations: Stories of India, Tales of Hypnosis*. Chicago: Chicago University Press.

Sil, Narasingha Prosad. 1997. *Swami Vivekananda: A Reassessment*. Selinsgrove, PA: Susquehanna University Press.

Sinclair, Upton. 1930. *Mental Radio*. Springfield, IL: Charles C. Thomas.

Singer, Milton B. 1972. *When a Great Tradition Modernizes: An Anthropological Approach to Indian Civilization.* New York: Praeger.

Singleton, Mark. 2005. "Salvation through Relaxation: Proprioceptive Therapy and Its Relationship to Yoga." *Journal of Contemporary Religion* 20 (3): 289–304.

Singleton, Mark. 2007a. "Suggestive Therapeutics: New Thought's Relationship to Modern Yoga." *Asian Medicine* 3: 64–84.

Singleton, Mark. 2007b. "Yoga, Eugenics, and Spiritual Darwinism in the Early Twentieth Century." *International Journal of Hindu Studies* 11 (2): 125–46.

Singleton, Mark. 2008. "The Classical Reveries of Modern Yoga." In *Yoga in the Modern World: Contemporary Perspectives*, edited by Mark Singleton and Jean Byrne, 77–99. New York: Routledge.

Singleton, Mark. 2010. *Yoga Body: The Origins of Modern Posture Practice.* New York: Oxford University Press.

Singleton, Mark, and Jean Byrne. 2008. "Introduction." In *Yoga in the Modern World: Contemporary Perspectives*, edited by Mark Singleton and Jean Byrne, 1–14. New York: Routledge.

Singleton, Mark, and Ellen Goldberg, eds. 2014. *Gurus of Modern Yoga.* New York: Oxford University Press.

Sloan, Mersene Elon. 1929. *The Indian Menace: An Essay of Exposure and Warning Showing the Strange Work of Hindu Propaganda in America and Its Special Danger to Our Women.* Washington, DC: Way Press.

Smith, Benjamin Richard. 2007. "Body, Mind and Spirit: Towards an Analysis of the Practice of Yoga." *Body & Society* 13 (2): 25–46.

Smith, Frederick M. 2006. *The Self Possessed: Deity and Spirit Possession in South Asian Literature and Civilization.* New York: Columbia University Press.

Sohi, Seema. 2014. *Echoes of Mutiny: Race, Surveillance, and Indian Anticolonialism in North America.* New York: Oxford University Press.

Stephens, Mark. 2010. *Teaching Yoga: Essential Foundations and Techniques.* Berkeley, CA: North Atlantic Books.

Stewart, Balfour, and P. G. Tait. 1875. *The Unseen Universe or Physical Speculations on a Future State.* New York: Macmillan.

Strauss, Sarah. 2005. *Positioning Yoga: Balancing Acts across Cultures.* New York: Berg.

Susman, Jordan. 2005. "Your Karma Ran Over My Dogma—Bikram Yoga and the (IM)Possibilities of Copyrighting Yoga." *Loyola of Los Angeles Entertainment Law Review* 25 (2): 245–74.

Syman, Stefanie. 2010. *The Subtle Body: The Story of Yoga in America.* New York: Farrar, Straus and Giroux.

Tesla, Nikola. 1930. "Man's Greatest Achievement." *New York American*, July 6.

Tesla, Nikola. 2011. *My Inventions and Other Writings.* Edited by Samantha Hunt. New York: Penguin Books.

The Washington Post. 1910. "Wooed as a God." May 8.

The Washington Post. 1912. "American Women Victims of Hindu Mysticism." February 12.

Thomas, Wendell Marshall. 1930. *Hinduism Invades America.* New York: Beacon Press.

Thoreau, Henry David. 2004. *Letters to a Spiritual Seeker.* Edited by Bradley P. Dean. New York: W. W. Norton.

Thursby, Gene R. 1995. "Hindu Movements since Mid-Century: Yogis in the States." In *America's Alternative Religions,* edited by Timothy Miller, 191–214. Albany: State University of New York Press.

Time. 1947. "Here Comes the Yogiman."

Törzsök, Judit. 1999. "The Doctrine of Magical Female Spirits: A Critical Edition of Selected Chapters of the Siddhayogeśvarīmata." D.Phil. thesis, Oxford University.

Treitel, Corinna. 2004. *A Science for the Soul: Occultism and the Genesis of the German Modern.* Baltimore: Johns Hopkins University Press.

Trine, Ralph Waldo. 1897. *In Tune with the Infinite; or, Fullness of Peace, Power, and Plenty.* New York: Thomas Y. Crowell.

Trout, Polly. 2000. *Eastern Seeds, Western Soil: Three Gurus in America.* Mountain View, CA: Mayfield Publishing Company.

Turner, Bryan S. 1994. *Orientalism, Postmodernism, and Globalism.* London: Routledge.

Tweed, Thomas A., and Stephen R. Prothero, eds. 1999. *Asian Religions in America: A Documentary History.* New York: Oxford University Press.

Urban, Hugh B. 2003. *Tantra: Sex, Secrecy, Politics, and Power in the Study of Religion.* Berkeley: University of California Press.

Van der Veer, Peter. 2001. *Imperial Encounters: Religion and Modernity in India and Britain.* Princeton: Princeton University Press.

Versluis, Arthur. 1993. *American Transcendentalism and Asian Religions.* New York: Oxford University Press.

Vivekananda, Swami. 1915. *The Complete Works of Swami Vivekananda.* Vol. 1. Calcutta: Advaita Ashrama.

Vivekananda, Swami. 1966. *The Complete Works of Swami Vivekananda.* Vol. 4. Calcutta: Advaita Ashrama.

Vivekananda, Swami. 1989a. *The Complete Works of Swami Vivekananda.* Vol. 5. Calcutta: Advaita Ashrama.

Vivekananda, Swami. 1989b. *The Complete Works of Swami Vivekananda.* Vol. 9. Calcutta: Advaita Ashrama.

Walker, Steven. 1983. "Vivekananda and American Occultism." In *The Occult in America: New Historical Perspectives,* edited by Howard Kerr and Charles L. Crow, 162–76. Urbana: University of Illinois Press.

Walters, J. Donald. 1967. *Yoga Postures for Higher Awareness.* Nevada City, CA: Crystal Clarity Publishers.

Walters, J. Donald. 1976. *Stories of Mukunda: True Episodes from the Boyhood of the Great Master Paramahansa Yogananda.* Nevada City, CA: Ananda Publications.

Walters, J. Donald. 2004. *Conversations with Yogananda*. Nevada City, CA: Crystal Clarity Publishers.

Warnack, James M. 1932. "Who Are the Swamis?" *Los Angeles Times*, December 25.

Washington, Peter. 1995. *Madame Blavatsky's Baboon: A History of the Mystics, Mediums, and Misfits Who Brought Spiritualism to America*. New York: Schocken Books.

Wassan, Yogi. 1939. *Secrets of the Himalaya Mountain Masters and Ladder to Cosmic Consciousness*. Denver, CO: C. B. Kimball.

Wessinger, Catherine, ed. 1993. *Women's Leadership in Marginal Religions: Explorations outside the Mainstream*. Urbana: University of Illinois Press.

Wessinger, Catherine. 1995. "Hinduism Arrives in America: The Vedanta Movement and the Self-Realization Fellowship." In *America's Alternative Religions*, edited by Timothy Miller, 173–90. Albany: State University of New York Press.

White, David Gordon. 1984. "Why Gurus Are Heavy." *Numen* 31 (1): 40–73.

White, David Gordon. 1996. *The Alchemical Body: Siddha Traditions in Medieval India*. Chicago: Chicago University Press.

White, David Gordon. 2002. *The Kiss of the Yoginī: Tantric Sex" in Its South Asian Contexts*. Chicago: University of Chicago Press.

White, David Gordon. 2009. *Sinister Yogis*. Chicago: University of Chicago Press.

White, David Gordon, ed. 2012. *Yoga in Practice*. Princeton: Princeton University Press.

White, David Gordon. 2014. *The Yoga Sutra of Patanjali: A Biography*. Princeton: Princeton University Press.

White, R. Andrew. 2006. "Stanislavsky and Ramacharaka: The Influence of Yoga and Turn-of-the-Century Occultism on the System." *Theatre Survey* 47 (1): 73–92.

Wilber, Ken, ed. 1984. *Quantum Questions: Mystical Writings of the World's Great Physicists*. New York: Random House.

Wildman, Sarah. 2011. "Kafka's Calisthenics: Watch and Learn the Favorite Exercise Routine of Early 20th Century Europeans." *Slate*, January 21. http://www.slate.com/articles/life/fitness/2011/01/kafkas_calisthenics.single.html.

Williamson, Lola. 2010. *Transcendent in America: Hindu-Inspired Meditation Movements as New Religion*. New York: New York University Press.

Winter, Alison. 1998. *Mesmerized: Powers of Mind in Victorian Britain*. Chicago: University of Chicago Press.

X, Mme. 1920. "Gymnastics after Dinner Mark True Follower of Yogi." *Chicago Daily Tribune*, August 8.

"Yoga in America Study." 2016. *Yoga Journal*. January 13. http://media.yogajournal.com/wp-content/uploads/2016-Yoga-in-America-Study-Comprehensive-RESULTS.pdf.

Yogananda, Paramahansa. 1946. *Autobiography of a Yogi*. New York: Philosophical Library.

Yogananda, Paramahansa. 1951. *Autobiography of a Yogi*. New York: Philosophical Library.

Yogananda, Paramahansa. 1954. *Autobiography of a Yogi*. Los Angeles: Self-Realization Fellowship.

Yogananda, Paramahansa. 1958. *Paramahansa Yogananda: In Memoriam: The Master's Life, Work, and Mahasamadhi*. Los Angeles: Self-Realization Fellowship.

Yogananda, Paramahansa. 1986. *The Divine Romance: Collected Talks and Essays on Realizing God in Daily Life*. Los Angeles: Self-Realization Fellowship.

Yogananda, Paramahansa. 1995. *Autobiography of a Yogi*. Nevada City, CA: Crystal Clarity Publishers.

Yogananda, Paramahansa. 1999. *God Talks with Arjuna: The Bhagavad Gita: Royal Science of God-Realization: The Immortal Dialogue Between Soul and Spirit*. Los Angeles: Self-Realization Fellowship.

Yogananda, Swami. 1923. *Songs of the Soul*. Boston: Sat Sanga.

Yogananda, Swami. 1925a. "History of Swami Yogananda's Work in America." *East-West* 1 (1): 7–11.

Yogananda, Swami. 1925b. *Yogoda or Tissue-Will System of Physical Perfection*. 5th ed. Boston: Sat-Sanga.

Yogananda, Swami. 1926a. "Miracles of Raja Yoga, Its Western Misconceptions." *East-West* 2 (2): 3–4.

Yogananda, Swami. 1926b. "Spiritualizing Business— Henry Ford's Five Day Working Week." *East-West* 2 (1): 3–4.

Yogananda, Swami. 1926c. "Who Is a Yogi?" *East-West* 1 (2): 15.

Yogananda, Swami. 1927. "Hamid Bey, 'Miracle Man.'" *East-West* 2 (6): 23–24.

Yogananda, Swami. 1928. *The Science of Religion*. Los Angeles: Yogoda Sat-Sanga Society.

Yogananda, Swami, and Swami Dhirananda. 1928. *Yogoda or Tissue-Will System of Physical Perfection*. 9th ed. Los Angeles: Yogoda Sat-Sanga Society.

"Yogoda Satsanga Society of India." 2015. http://www.yssofindia.org.

Index